WALKING
SEATTLE

35 tours of the Jet City's parks, landmarks, neighborhoods, and scenic views

Clark Humphrey

 WILDERNESS PRESS ... *on the trail since 1967*

Walking Seattle: 35 tours of the Jet City's parks, landmarks, neighborhoods, and scenic views

1st EDITION 2011
  2nd printing 2014

Front cover photos copyright © 2011 by the author
Interior photos, except where noted, by the author
Maps: Author and Scott McGrew
Interior and cover design: Larry Van Dyke and Scott McGrew
Layout: Annie Long
Editor: Laura Shauger

ISBN 978-0-89997-498-9

Manufactured in the United States of America

Published by: Wilderness Press
                Keen Communications
                P.O. Box 43673
                Birmingham, AL 35243
                (800) 443-7227; FAX (205) 326-1012
                info@wildernesspress.com
                www.wildernesspress.com

Visit our website for a complete listing of our books and for ordering information.
Distributed by Publishers Group West

Cover photos: *Front, clockwise from upper right:* Fishermen's memorial, Myrtle Edwards Park; Space Needle from Fisher Plaza; Green Lake; Pike Place Market main entrance; Central Library; Experience Music Project, Seattle Center; downtown skyline from Magnolia. *Back, top to bottom:* Washington State Convention Center skybridge; Old Pequliar Alehouse, Ballard; Alki Point lighthouse.

SAFETY NOTICE: Although Wilderness Press and the author have made every attempt to ensure that the information in this book is accurate at press time, they are not responsible for any loss, damage, injury, or inconvenience that may occur to anyone while using this book. Always check local conditions, know your own limitations, and consult a map.

acknowledgments

Roslyn Bullas originally hired me to write this book. Gregory Zura first suggested I pursue it.

Many, many people helped me decide what local attractions absolutely had to get included here. A few of them include Revele Kelley, Laura Castellanos, Kurt Geissel, Marlow Harris, Elaine Bonow, Patricia Devine, Julie Pheasant-Albright, Shawn Wolfe, Missy Chow, Bill Shaw, and Mark Harlow.

author's note

There's so much to see and do in Seattle. My hardest job was devising only 35 routes that would include most of the city's natural and built attractions. Some of the places that didn't fit are mentioned in sidebars.

Even within the neighborhoods I do cover, space requirements meant I had to leave out a lot of cool places. If you've got the time, go ahead and stray from the written path. Just be sure you can retrace your steps back.

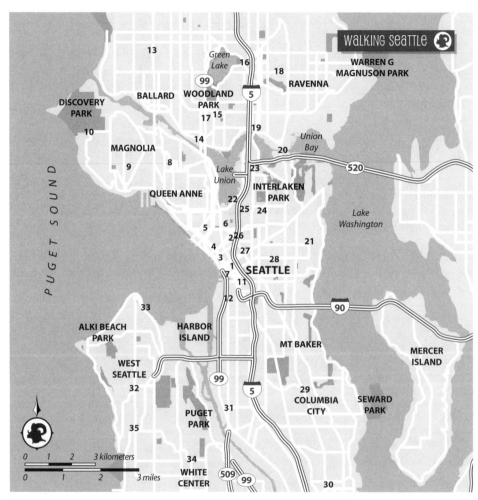

WALKING SEATTLE

NUMBERS ON THIS LOCATOR MAP CORRESPOND TO WALK NUMBERS.

TaBLE OF CONTENTS

INTRODUCTION

Seattle. Jet City. Portal of the North Pacific. Queen City of the Pacific Northwest. "Metronatural" (to use a recent tourist slogan). The "Emerald City" (to quote a previous tourist slogan). Land of airplanes, software, coffee, fish, casual wear, and indie rock bands.

Whatever you call it, it's a young city with a lot of history. Once a frontier settlement at the nation's far corner, it's now a crossroads of world trade and cultures.

And it's a great place to walk. We've got lush greenery. We've got mountain and water views. We've got cozy bungalows, stately mansions, postmodern palaces, and outdoor art all over. We've got wide boulevards, narrow cobblestone lanes, and carless pedestrian pathways. It seldom gets too cold to go walking, and almost never gets too hot.

Seattle is a wonderful walking city. Just be careful of the hills. We've got some steep ones here, even after the massive pre-World War I regrading projects. When possible, I've devised these walks to avoid the more punishing inclines. The one exception, in Discovery Park (Walk 10), can be taken in reverse to avoid the steepest climb.

I've walked every foot of these trips, most of them several times, in different seasons. Each one will take you on an adventure through one of the most fascinating cityscapes in the United States.

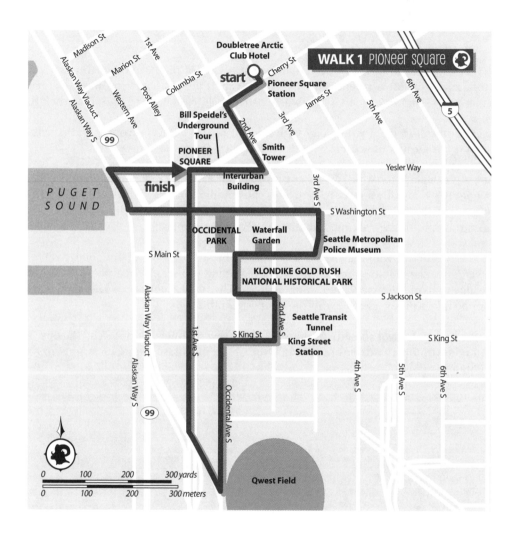

WALK 1 PIONEER SQUARE

Madison St

1st Ave

Marion St

Alaskan Way Viaduct

Alaskan Way S

99

Western Ave

Post Alley

Columbia St

Doubletree Arctic Club Hotel

start

Cherry St

Pioneer Square Station

James St

3rd Ave

5th Ave

6th Ave

5

2nd Ave

Bill Speidel's Underground Tour

PIONEER SQUARE

Smith Tower

finish

Interurban Building

PUGET SOUND

3rd Ave S

Yesler Way

S Washington St

OCCIDENTAL PARK

Waterfall Garden

Seattle Metropolitan Police Museum

S Main St

KLONDIKE GOLD RUSH NATIONAL HISTORICAL PARK

S Jackson St

Alaskan Way Viaduct

1st Ave S

S King St

2nd Ave S

Seattle Transit Tunnel

King Street Station

S King St

Alaskan Way S

99

Occidental Ave S

4th Ave S

5th Ave S

6th Ave S

Qwest Field

0   100   200   300 yards
0   100   200   300 meters

1 Pioneer Square: Where Seattle Started

BOUNDARIES: **3rd Ave., Cherry St., 1st Ave. S., and Qwest Field**
DISTANCE: **1¾ miles**
DIFFICULTY: **Easy (all flat or downhill)**
PARKING: **Limited metered street parking; pay lots and garages**
PUBLIC TRANSIT: **Seattle Transit Tunnel Pioneer Square Station, 3rd Ave. south of Cherry St.;
    numerous Metro bus routes on 3rd**

The first white settlement in present-day Seattle was established in 1851 at Alki Point (Walk 33). After one miserable winter there, the settlers built a township along a small patch of level land surrounded by forested hills, tidal flats, and Elliott Bay. This is where Henry Yesler built his lumber mill, where the logs for Yesler's mill were skidded downhill on the original "skid road," where the first stores, saloons, and bawdy houses opened. Those wooden buildings burned in the Great Seattle Fire of 1889. They were replaced by brick and stone structures, advertisements of a town striving for greatness. These architectural classics were preserved by neglect as downtown's core moved north. They're now mostly intact and restored as monuments to yesterday's hopes for a grand tomorrow.

● **Start at the Doubletree Arctic Club Hotel, 700 3rd Ave.** This stoic white-clad structure was built in 1916 by business leaders associated with the Alaska trade. The building notes this connection with rows of terra-cotta walrus heads, whose tusks were originally marble (since replaced with terra-cotta and plastic). The club's meeting space was the grand Dome Room, named for its curved stained-glass ceiling. The building's now an elegant boutique hotel, and the Dome Room is its lounge and dining area. Walk southeast from here to Cherry St.

● **Cross 3rd at Cherry.** In front of you is the Dexter Horton Building, another terra-cotta palace. It was built in 1924 for the Dexter Horton National Bank, which merged with two other banks in the 1930s to become Seattle-First National Bank (Walk 3). On the southwest side of Cherry stands the Lyon Building, six handsome stories of brick and concrete dating to 1910. Walk on the northwest side of Cherry to 2nd Ave. Across 2nd is the 18-story, Beaux Arts Hoge Building, Seattle's tallest building when it was built in 1911.

- Turn southeast on 2nd. Enjoy the terra-cotta angels, serpents, and torches embellishing the Alaska Building. In 1904 it was Seattle's first steel-frame skyscraper (14 stories). Across 2nd is the Broderick Building (623 2nd Ave.), one of the original stone structures built after the 1889 fire. To its left, a parking garage incorporates the ground-floor facade of the 1893 Butler Hotel. Continue on 2nd past three smaller old buildings to the Smith Tower.

  When typewriter tycoon L. C. Smith built it in 1914, the Smith Tower was the tallest building west of the Mississippi. It remained Seattle's tallest until 1962. Its white base is topped by a smaller tower section, and then by a pyramid-shaped cap. The pyramid's base (the building's 35th floor) is the Chinese Room, a lavish space available for rentals (or simply for enjoying inside and outside views). The building also features marble-and-brass interiors and Seattle's last old-time steam elevators, with professional operators.

- Turn west on Yesler, the original "Skid Road," where logs were skidded downhill toward Henry Yesler's sawmill, and continue for two blocks. (Note: Yesler, and the streets south of it, are on a north-south grid. Downtown streets north of Yesler run parallel to the waterfront, on a northwest-southeast grid.) Immediately west of the Smith Tower is the infamous "sinking ship" parking garage, built in 1963 on the venerable 1889 Seattle Hotel's site. A few years later, developers proposed razing most of the neighborhood for more parking. Instead, preservationists got Pioneer Square declared a historic district.

  On Yesler's south side are the 1892 Interurban Building and the 1890 Merchants Cafe (still open as a restaurant after 120 years). On its north side, the stoic 1892 Pioneer Building is home to the Underground Tour, founded in the 1980s by entrepreneur-historian Bill Speidel. The guided tour traverses the original ground floors of the square buildings, turned into basements when the street levels were raised.

  The Pioneer Building overlooks Pioneer Square itself, a.k.a. Pioneer Place Park. This cobblestoned triangle was established in 1893 on the former site of Yesler's mill. An Alaskan totem pole was added in 1899; it burned, and a new pole was commissioned, in 1938. The ornate iron pergola facing Yesler was built in 1909 (and rebuilt twice since); it was originally a trolley-stop shelter and an entrance to now-closed underground restrooms.

- Turn south on 1st Ave. S. In the late 19th and early 20th century lumberjacks and farm boys cavorted in saloons and brothels in this "Great Restricted District." In the 1970s, this street took on a double life—galleries and boutiques by day, raucous bars by night. Both scenes slumped in the late 2000s but survive, as do the vintage brick buildings. Toward this segment's end is Sluggers Bar & Grill, which claims to be the first TV-festooned sports bar in the United States.

- Turn southeast on the diagonal Railroad Way S. to Occidental Ave. S. You're facing the west side of Qwest Field, one of two luxurious stadia that replaced the utilitarian Kingdome. Qwest hosts the NFL's Seahawks, Major League Soccer's Sounders FC, concerts, and boat and home shows.

- Turn north on Occidental, abutting Qwest Field's parking lot. To your left is the Florentine (526 1st Ave. S.), a condo and retail structure built from a really long 1909 warehouse. Occidental doglegs at S. King St. in front of F. X. McRory's, which was a luxurious sports bar even during the humbler Kingdome era.

- Turn east on S. King. To your right looms Qwest Field's north entrance, featuring artist Bob Haozous's *Earth Dialogue,* four disk-shaped silhouettes representing humanity's connection to the natural world. Ahead of you lies King Street Station, built in 1906. Its 242-foot clock tower was inspired by Venice's Campanile di San Marco. It now services Amtrak and commuter rail. Its once-grand waiting room is being restored.

- Turn north from King onto 2nd Ave. S. To your right, a new King County office building strives to fit in with its historic surroundings. To your left, the Court in the Square is a glass-ceilinged atrium between two brick buildings.

- Turn west onto S. Jackson St. To your right, the historic Cadillac Hotel now houses the Klondike Gold Rush National Historical Park, a free museum about the 1897 Yukon gold fever that helped put Seattle on the map. To your left, Zeitgeist Kunst & Kaffee is a handsome, retro-industrial space. Beyond it stands the 1903 Washington Shoe Building, a factory that later became art studios and now hosts offices.

Back Story: Seattle's Street System

Seattle's street naming system is really easy once you know the basic rules (which have their exceptions). Streets generally run east-west; in greater downtown (including Belltown and west Capitol Hill), they run northeast-southwest. Avenues generally run north-south; in greater downtown, they run northwest-southeast. Ways, drives, places, boulevards, etc. can run in any direction.

Downtown's not the only place where the city's geography inspired digressions from an orderly street grid. Just about every part of town has them. These walks routinely cross the city's directional prefix and suffix zones (NW, N., NE, etc.). Don't worry about it.

Central downtown's streets were given alliterative pairs of names for easier remembering—Jefferson and James, Columbia and Cherry, Marion and Madison, Spring and Seneca, University and Union, and Pike and Pine. These are expressed in an old-time local phrase, "Jesus Christ Made Seattle Under Protest."

- Walk north through Occidental Mall. This pedestrian-only corridor abuts several fine art galleries, and serves as a more intimate counterpart to Occidental Park, the next block north. The latter features two large totem poles and the *Fallen Firefighter Memorial* statues.

- Turn east on S. Main St. At the southeast corner of 2nd and Main, the 1929 Seattle Fire Department headquarters stands as a stony symbol of stoic dedication. At the northwest corner of 2nd and Main, the Waterfall Garden Park is a small enclosed outdoor space in front of an artificial waterfall. It was built in 1977 by the family that founded the formerly Seattle-based United Parcel Service. Farther along, a gyro stand occupies a vintage gas station at the intersection with the diagonal 2nd Ave. Extension. The northeast corner of 3rd and Main offers more major commercial art galleries.

● Turn north on 3rd Ave. S. Halfway up the block, the privately run Seattle Metropolitan Police Museum claims to be the largest police museum in the western United States. At the southwest corner of 3rd and Washington, the 1890 Washington Court Building was originally commissioned by Dorothea "Lou" Graham, early Seattle's most famous brothel operator. It's now part of the Union Gospel Mission. At the northeast corner, the Tashiro/Kaplan Building combines two vintage structures into artist studios and galleries.

● Turn west on S. Washington St. for five blocks. At the northeast corner of Washington and the 2nd Ave. Extension, the three-story 1890 Chin Gee Hee Building is the last vestige of Seattle's original Chinatown, before that community gradually moved farther east (Walk 11). At this intersection's northwest corner, the Nugent/Considine Block houses the Double Header Tavern, Seattle's oldest gay bar. In that building's basement, the Heaven Nightclub occupies vaudeville mogul John Considine's People's Theater. One block beyond, the historic buildings give way to the 1950s brutalism of the Alaskan Way Viaduct (Walk 7). Beyond this, at the foot of Alaskan Way, stands the Washington Street Boat Landing, a Beaux Arts metal pergola built in 1920.

● Turn northwest on Alaskan one block; then turn east on Yesler. The 1914 Pioneer Square Hotel and Saloon has been renovated as a boutique hotel. Back at 1st and Yesler, the red sandstone facade of the Mutual Life Building now sports a toy store.

CONNECTING THE WALKS

This walk starts one block southwest of Walk 2, and it ends near Walks 3, 4, and 7. At Railroad and Occidental you're one block north of Walk 12. At 2nd and Jackson you're three blocks west and one block north of Walk 11.

POINTS OF INTEREST

Doubletree Arctic Club Hotel doubletree.hilton.com, 700 3rd Ave., 206-340-0340

Smith Tower smithtower.com, 506 2nd Ave., 206-622-4004

Bill Speidel's Underground Tour undergroundtour.com, 608 1st Ave., 206-682-4646

Pioneer Square seattle.gov/parks, 1st Ave. and Yesler Way

Qwest Field qwestfield.com, 800 Occidental Ave. S., 206-682-2900

King Street Station seattle.gov/transportation/kingstreet.htm, 303 S. Jackson St., 206-382-4125

Klondike Gold Rush National Historical Park nps.gov/klse, 319 2nd Ave. S., 206-220-4240

Occidental Park seattle.gov/parks, Occidental Ave. S. and S. Washington St.

Waterfall Garden Park 219 2nd Ave. S.

Seattle Metropolitan Police Museum seametropolicemuseum.org, 317 3rd Ave. S., 206-748-9991

route summary

1. Start at the Doubletree Arctic Club Hotel, 700 3rd Ave. Walk southeast on 3rd.
2. Turn southwest on Cherry St.
3. Turn southeast on 2nd Ave.
4. Turn west on Yesler Way to Pioneer Square.
5. Turn south on 1st Ave. S.
6. Turn southeast on Railroad Way S. to Qwest Field.
7. Turn north on Occidental Ave. S.
8. Turn east on S. King St.
9. Turn north on 2nd Ave. S.
10. Turn west on S. Jackson St.
11. Turn north through Occidental Mall and Occidental Park.
12. Turn east on S. Main St.
13. Turn north on 3rd Ave S.
14. Turn west on S. Washington St.
15. Turn northwest on Alaskan Way S.
16. Turn east on Yesler, back to 1st Ave.

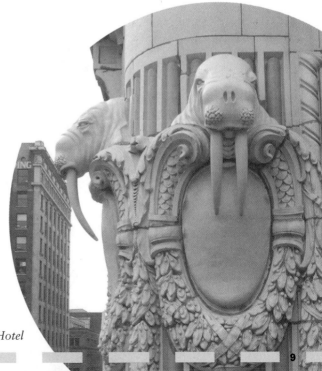

Terra-cotta walrus heads at the Doubletree Arctic Club Hotel

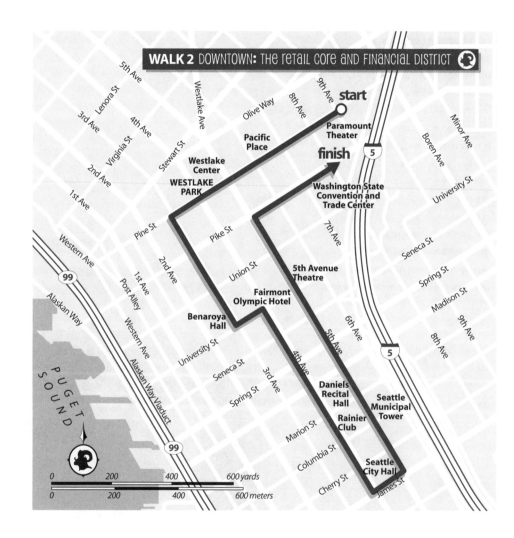

WALK 2 DOWNTOWN: The retail core and financial district

start

Paramount Theater

finish

Pacific Place

Westlake Center

WESTLAKE PARK

Washington State Convention and Trade Center

5th Avenue Theatre

Fairmont Olympic Hotel

Benaroya Hall

Daniels Recital Hall

Rainier Club

Seattle Municipal Tower

Seattle City Hall

PUGET SOUND

5th Ave
Lenora St
3rd Ave
4th Ave
Virginia St
2nd Ave
1st Ave
Westlake Ave
Stewart St
Olive Way
8th Ave
9th Ave
Minor Ave
Boren Ave
University St
Pine St
Pike St
7th Ave
Seneca St
Spring St
Madison St
9th Ave
8th Ave
2nd Ave
Union St
Western Ave
1st Ave
Post Alley
Alaskan Way
Western Ave
University St
Seneca St
Spring St
3rd Ave
4th Ave
5th Ave
6th Ave
Marion St
Columbia St
Cherry St
James St
Alaskan Way Viaduct

99
99
5
5

0   200   400   600 yards
0   200   400   600 meters

2 DOWNTOWN: THe reTaiL core anD FinanciaL DisTricT: skyscrapers anD SHOPPING

BOUNDARIES: 9th Ave., Pine St., 3rd Ave., and James St.
DISTANCE: 2 miles
DIFFICULTY: Moderate (one uphill block)
PARKING: Limited metered street parking; pay lots and garages include Pacific Place Garage (6th Ave. north of Pine St).
PUBLIC TRANSIT: Seattle Transit Tunnel Convention Place Station, 9th Ave. and Pine Street; Metro routes #10, 11, 14, 43, and 49 serve Pike and Pine streets.

Seattle is blessed to have an active, dynamic downtown that never succumbed to the urban decay faced by other cities around the United States. It might not be a 24-hour place, but it's at least a 16-hour place. And it's devoted to more than the mere making and spending of money. It offers a wide range of live and filmed entertainments. It has a major art museum and many private galleries. It has occasional peekaboo views of the Elliott Bay waterfront and the Olympic Mountains. And as you're about to see, it sports an array of architectural styles, from 1920s deco whimsy to postmodern color play and angularity.

● **Start at the Paramount Theater,** on the southeast corner of 9th Ave. and Pine St. Seattle's master theater designer B. Marcus Priteca helped create this sumptuous 1928 film-and-vaudeville palace, with a handsome brick exterior and a Versailles-inspired interior. The blue vertical sign outside is a 2009 copy of the original. Looking northwest on 9th, you can see the rooftop Gothic neon announcing the 1926-built Camlin Hotel, now part of a time-share circuit.

● **Go southwest on Pine.** At the southeast corner of 8th and Pine, the cylindrical Tower 801 apartment building houses a retro-modern Caffe Ladro coffeehouse at its base. Kitty-corner from there, the Paramount Hotel's Dragonfish bar offers happy hour sushi bites and a wall of silent pachinko machines. At 7th, midcentury-esque bar and grill Von's anchors the 1929 Roosevelt Hotel.

Back Story: renamed Buildings

Many local buildings have gone through name changes because of acquisitions, rebranding, and other motivations. Many old-timers insist on using the buildings' previous names. Here's a guide to the more prominent renamings:

NOW	THEN
Nordstrom	Frederick & Nelson
Macy's	The Bon Marché
Safeco Plaza	1000 4th Avenue Plaza; Seafirst Tower
UW Tower (U District)	Safeco Plaza
Russell Investments Center	WaMu Center
Fairmont Olympic Hotel	Four Seasons Olympic; The Olympic
UW Plaza (Fourth Ave.)	Puget Sound Plaza
US Bank Centre	City Centre; Pacific First Centre
1201 Third Avenue	Washington Mutual Tower
Wells Fargo Center	First Interstate Center
Seattle Municipal Tower	AT&T Gateway Tower; Key Bank Tower
Columbia Center	Bank of America Tower; Columbia Seafirst Center
Qwest Plaza	1600 Bell Plaza; US West Building; Pacific Northwest Bell Building

● Cross Pine at the southeast corner with 7th Ave. toward the Pacific Place mall. Opened in 1998, it's a single full-block building disguised with a variety of false facades. Within, upscale chain stores and a multiplex cinema surround a four-story atrium. Across 6th, the Nordstrom flagship store and headquarters building (a handsome white 1918 structure) was remodeled in 1998 from the former Frederick & Nelson, a classy (and still missed) department store that folded in 1992.

On the next block, the Westlake Center mall and office tower was built a decade before Pacific Place, when Seattle's business leaders were less obsessed with high-end luxury everything. Pacific Place has Tiffany's and the Italian-bistro chain Il Fornaio; Westlake Center has Hot Topic and a Sbarro pizza stand. Across Pine from Westlake Center, triangular Westlake Park is the site of high-profile political rallies and commercial publicity events.

At the northwest side of 4th is Seattle's other heritage department store, built in 1928 as The Bon Marché. It now bears the Macy's brand, but old-timers still call it "the Bon." Like the Frederick & Nelson (now Nordstrom) building, it gained four stories in the 1950s. You can tell where the newer part starts—the terra-cotta becomes a lot simpler.

● Turn southeast on 3rd Ave. Near Pike St. is the Century Square retail and office complex (known to some as "the Braun shaver building" for its curved roof). Across Pike stand the onetime outposts of five-and-dime rivals Woolworth and Kress. The former now houses Ross Dress for Less; the latter's tenants include an IGA supermarket (in the basement). At Union St., a cinema that went porno in the '70s is now the Triple Door, a posh music and cabaret joint. Beyond Union is the swank Benaroya Hall, home of the Seattle Symphony. It looks a lot like a streamlined modern Protestant church—if Protestant churches had huge Dale Chihuly chandeliers in their lobbies.

● Turn northeast on University St. On the southeast corner of 3rd and University, the 1929 Seattle (née Northern Life) Tower is a 27-story art deco mountain peak. (We'll look more closely at it in Walk 3.) At this intersection's northwest corner, the 1910 Cobb Building is 11 stories of Beaux Arts brick cladding with a graceful curved corner. Its former full-block-long clone across 4th, the White-Henry-Stuart Building, was razed in the 1970s for Rainier Square, a glass-and-steel tower above an odd, tapered pedestal above-ground-floor retail. It was designed by Seattle architect Minoru Yama-saki, who also designed the World Trade Center towers in New York.

- Cross 4th Ave. and walk southeast. To your left, the 1924 Olympic Hotel remains, as an old ad slogan put it, "the hotel Seattle calls home." Once the flagship of the chain now known as Westin, it's now run by the Toronto-based Fairmont Hotels. On the following block, three newer hotels offer less-formal luxury lodgings. Beyond Spring St. two buildings, the Seattle Central Library and Safeco Plaza, bookend four decades of monumental architecture (more about them in Walk 3).

- To your left south of Madison St. stands the 901 Fifth Avenue Building, built in 1974 for the Bank of California; the Bartell Drug store on the ground floor used to be that bank's lobby. At the end of that block, the YMCA's collegiate Gothic–style building was a 1931 addition to the 1907 original, since razed for an office tower. To your right beyond Marion St., the Pacific (née Leamington) Hotel, a pair of 1918 low-rises, has been respectfully altered into affordable apartments. To your left from there, the ivy-covered Rainier Club has been the city's poshest private meeting and dining hall since 1904. One block farther, across Columbia St., the three concave towers of Columbia Center rise 76 stories, the tallest building west of the Mississippi.

- Continue on 4th beyond Cherry St. to the 2003-vintage City Hall, a grand postmodern space with a two-level public square. A Nordic-modern City Council chamber anchors its interior. If you're walking during regular business hours, you can take City Hall's elevators up to its 5th Ave. level and out its eastern exit. Otherwise, take a steep walk up James St., past the King County Administration Building (which looks a lot like an old console TV set with the doors closed).

- Turn northwest on 5th Ave. The police department and municipal court are in the Seattle Justice Center at 5th and James. The city bought an entire high-rise from a bankrupt developer; it's now the Seattle Municipal Tower beyond Cherry St. At the southwest corner of 5th and Marion, Daniels Recital Hall occupies a grand 1908 Beaux Arts building, formerly First United Methodist Church.

Beyond Madison St., the 1940 Nakamura Federal Courthouse sits behind a half-block lawn that used to be downtown's biggest open space. Just before Seneca St., the

1913 YWCA building offers relief sculptures of classical Greek women reading scrolls and holding swords. Just across Seneca, the IBM Building is another Minoru Yama-saki design in understated white stripes and clean lines and curves.

North of University St., the Skinner Building somehow combines two 1920s styles, Mediterranean palazzo and Chinese exotica. The latter is most prevalent inside the building's anchor space, the 5th Avenue Theatre, another movie palace that now hosts stage musicals. (The big exterior sign is a new addition, designed to look as if it had always been there.)

To your right at 5th and Pike St., the US Bank Centre is a 1980s attempt to bring ornamental frills back to office-tower architecture. Across Pike, Banana Republic occupies what had been Priteca's 1916 Coliseum Theater, billed by some as the first US building made expressly as a movie house. On the intersection's northwest side, three former Nordstrom buildings now host Urban Outfitters and Sephora.

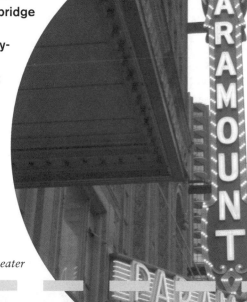

- Turn northeast (right) on Pike past a Sheraton hotel and recent chain-retail structures. Continue at 8th Ave., to a domed skybridge over Pike at the Washington State Convention and Trade Center. The sky-bridge wasn't there when the World Trade Organization met here in 1999; if it had been, thousands of street-filling protesters wouldn't have succeeded in blocking access to the place.

- To return to this walk's start, walk to 9th and Pine, then take a left and continue for one block.

Paramount Theater

CONNeCTING THe WaLKS

This walk connects easily to a half dozen other walks. It crosses Walk 3 at several points. It ends three blocks southwest of Walk 26. At 5th and Pine you're three blocks southeast of Walk 5. At 3rd and Pine you're two blocks from Walk 4. At 4th and Cherry you're one block northeast of Walk 1. At 5th and Seneca you're three blocks southwest of Walk 27.

POINTS OF INTeReST

Paramount Theater stgpresents.org, 911 Pine St., 206-467-5510

Pacific Place pacificplaceseattle.com, 600 Pine St.

Westlake Center westlakecenter.com, 400 Pine St.

Benaroya Hall seattlesymphony.org, 200 University St., 206-215-4800

Fairmont Olympic Hotel fairmont.com/seattle, 411 University St., 206-621-1700

Daniels Recital Hall recitalhall.fifthandcolumbia.com, 811 5th Ave., 425-922-6810

5th Avenue Theatre 5thavenue.org, 1326 5th Ave., 206-625-1900

Washington State Convention and Trade Center wsctc.com, 7th Ave. and Pike St.

rOUTe SUMMarY

1. Start at 9th Ave. and Pine St.
2. Go southwest on Pine to 7th Ave.
3. Cross Pine at 7th. Continue on Pine to 3rd Ave.
4. Turn southeast on 3rd.
5. Turn northeast on University St.
6. Turn onto 4th Ave. and walk southeast.
7. Turn northeast on James St., or cut through City Hall, to 5th Ave.
8. Turn northwest on 5th.
9. Turn northeast on Pike to 8th Ave.

King County Administration Building

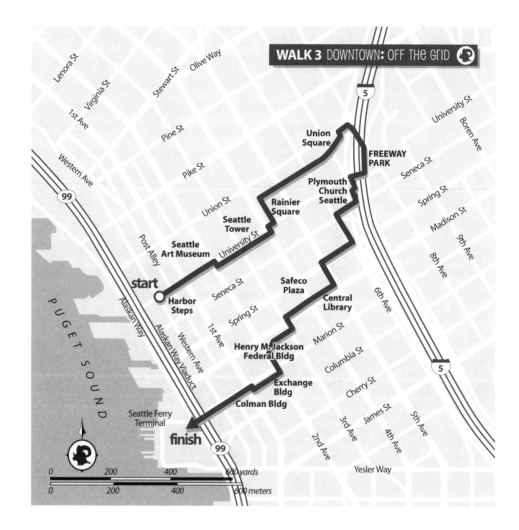

Lenora St
Virginia St
1st Ave
Stewart St
Olive Way
Pine St
Pike St
Western Ave
99
Union St
Seattle Tower
Post Alley
Seattle Art Museum
University St
Rainier Square
Union Square
Plymouth Church Seattle
FREEWAY PARK
5
University St
Boren Ave
Seneca St
Spring St
Madison St
9th Ave
8th Ave
start
Harbor Steps
Seneca St
Spring St
1st Ave
Alaskan Way
Western Ave
Alaskan Way Viaduct
Safeco Plaza
Central Library
6th Ave
Marion St
Henry M. Jackson Federal Bldg
Columbia St
Cherry St
James St
5th Ave
4th Ave
3rd Ave
2nd Ave
Exchange Bldg
Colman Bldg
Seattle Ferry Terminal
finish
99
5
Yesler Way

P U G E T   S O U N D

0   200   400   600 yards
0   200   400   600 meters

3 DOWNTOWN: OFF THE GRID: THE CITY CENTER, OFF-CENTER

BOUNDARIES: **Western Ave., Union St., Freeway Park, Alaskan Way, and Marion St.**
DISTANCE: **1½ miles**
DIFFICULTY: **Moderate (a few mild inclines)**
PARKING: **Limited metered street parking; pay lots and garages, including a lot at Western and University and a garage at Western and Seneca St.**
PUBLIC TRANSIT: **Metro routes #10, 11, 12, 15, 18, 21, 22, and 56 stop at 1st Ave. and University St.**

Downtown's spectacular vistas come with a price. Parts of it are almost too steep to walk. (Some side-street sidewalks are equipped with raised concrete ridges, to help prevent pedestrians from falling backward. Really.) Fortunately, there are ways to lessen this burden. City zoning has long encouraged property owners to add elevators, escalators, tunnels, and other amenities to help move people around the hardest hill climbs. All the shortcuts in this walk (including those on private property) are open to the public, at least during business hours. They also offer up-close and inside views of some of the city's most spectacular artificial spectacles, from Freeway Park's giant flower-box setting to the Seattle Tower's understated elegance to the Exchange Building's deco glamour.

● Start at Western Ave. and University St. A century ago, Western was the "Commission District," home to Seattle's wholesale produce industry. Now its warehouses have become loft offices. A whale mural by James Crespinel stands at the northwest corner of this intersection, on the Seattle Steam Co. plant (an independent central-heating provider). To your right are the Harbor Steps, a grand outdoor stairway straddling an office, condo, hotel, and retail complex. Climb these steps, or take the public elevator just south of University, to 1st Ave.

● Cross 1st at University's north side to the original (1991) end of the Seattle Art Museum, intended by architect Robert Venturi to resemble an upmarket version of a "decorated shed," albeit a shed clad in limestone and granite. Take the wide outdoor plaza steps to 2nd Ave. and cross.

Pay your respects to the region's war dead at the Garden of Remembrance, on the 2nd Ave. side of Benaroya Hall. Cross University to the northern entrance of the 1201 Third Avenue Building (formerly Washington Mutual Tower, the older of two towers built for that defunct bank). Take the escalator to, then exit through, the 3rd Ave. lobby.

● Cross 3rd and enter the Seattle Tower lobby, an art deco dreamscape in bronze and marble. Take the elevators to the fifth floor. There, take a right and leave through the alley skybridge to the plaza outside the Financial Center building. Descend that plaza's outdoor stairs.

● Cross kitty-corner at 4th and University, taking a gander at the Olympic Hotel and Cobb Building along the way (Walk 2). Take the south lobby entrance into Rainier Square's lobby. Once inside, turn right at the signs for the pedestrian concourse. This three-block-long underground passage connects to the Skinner Building, Seattle Hilton, and Washington Athletic Club. Its walls are lined with big posters chronicling the history of downtown Seattle and that of Seattle's onetime biggest employer, the Boeing Co.

● This concourse ends at a pair of escalators. Take the up escalator into Two Union Square's food court. Walk toward a small waiting area with a fireplace. Turn left. At your earliest opportunity, turn right. Take a shorter escalator up, into the building's upper lobby level. Walk straight and out the building, onto another skybridge.

● On this skybridge, take a left and admire the stately old Eagles Auditorium, now home to ACT (A Contemporary Theatre). It hosted acid-rock acts in the 1960s; despite popular legend, Jimi Hendrix never played there. Turn right and enter the Washington State Convention Center's second floor. Rotating public-art exhibits line its corridors.

● Take an escalator jaunt to the Convention Center's fourth floor. Walk straight from the escalator's end, toward a big glass wall. Take the glass doors to your left, out of the Convention Center and into Freeway Park. This labyrinth of landscaped concrete platforms predates the Convention Center by a decade. When Interstate 5 was routed between downtown and First Hill in the early 1960s, some citizens protested. They

Back Story: The WTO

In their eternal obsession with being seen as "a world class city," Seattle's civic leaders successfully lobbied to host the World Trade Organization's 1999 ministerial conference. Despite the presence of many Sixties Generation vets in the City Council and other official bodies, nobody seemed to think mass protests could occur against the WTO; even though it was widely reviled for, among other things, ordering national governments to change their laws to appease corporations.

On what the protesters called "N30" (November 30, 1999), more than 40,000 demonstrators took to the downtown streets, blocking Convention Center access. A smaller team of black-clothed anarchists, meanwhile, spray-painted and threw rocks at chain store windows. Police used pepper spray, tear gas, and rubber bullets to force the demonstrators out of the immediate area. The daylong Battle in Seattle was later fictionalized in a movie of the same name—mostly filmed in Vancouver, British Columbia.

called for a roof over the freeway, to keep the two neighborhoods connected. They got a small lid years later, in 1976.

- Walk straight ahead through Freeway Park. At the first path intersection, take a right-and-left dogleg. At the next intersection, take a hard right. Walk downhill to the park's tail end at the outdoor plaza of the Park Place tower, 6th Ave. and Seneca St.

- Cross kitty-corner at 6th and Seneca. At this intersection's northwest corner stands Plymouth Church Seattle, a stunning example of a modern Protestant church, all white and asymmetrical. At the southwest corner, the Holiday Inn Crowne Plaza Hotel's developers promised a public open space in return for getting to build a taller hotel. They built a tiny windswept plaza atop a very obscure flight of stairs (just try to find it). Go southeast on 6th one block to the University Women's Club, a brick Georgian Revival building.

- Turn southwest on Spring St., passing the Nakamura Courthouse. Turn southeast on 5th to the Seattle Central Library, a postmodern masterwork. Opened in 2004 and designed by Dutch architect Rem Koolhaas, its asymmetric "stacks" allow different square footage for different uses, leading to a spectacular reading room on the tenth floor. Enter at the library's southeast side. Take the escalator down to the first floor; exit the library at 4th Ave.

- Cross 4th at Madison St. to Safeco Plaza. This 50-story black box was Seattle's tallest building when built in 1968 (downtown's first big privately-funded building in nearly 40 years). It opened as the headquarters of Seattle-First National Bank, the state's largest bank until it decided to speculate in Oklahoma oil leases in the 1980s. Seafirst was sold to Bank of America for pennies on the dollar. The building's now headquarters to a homegrown insurance company, itself sold to Liberty Mutual. Pass Henry Moore's *Vertebrae* sculpture, enter the main lobby, take the elevators or escalators down, and exit onto 3rd Ave.

- Cross kitty-corner at 3rd and Madison. Walk through the lobby of the trapezoidal Wells Fargo Center. At its western end, take a covered outdoor escalator down to 2nd and Marion St.

- Cross kitty-corner at 2nd and Marion, passing the Henry M. Jackson Federal Building (with the entry arch and other pieces of the stone midrise it replaced, the Burke Building, now used as plaza art). At this intersection's southwest corner, the 1929 Exchange Building is another art deco masterpiece. Enter its dark marble lobby with a gilt ceiling; take its elevators to, and exit through, its 1st Ave. level.

- Cross 1st at Marion to the Colman Building. This block-long midrise was built in stages between 1889 and 1904, and has been remodeled several times since. Walk one block southwest on Marion back to Western, or take a skybridge at the Colman Building's north side to the Washington State Ferry Terminal.

CONNECTING THE WALKS

This walk connects easily to five other walks. It crosses Walk 2 at several points, starts and ends two blocks northeast of Walk 7, and crosses Walk 4 at 1st Ave. At 1st and Marion you're three blocks northwest of Walk 1. At 6th and Seneca you're two blocks southeast of Walk 27.

POINTS OF INTEREST

Harbor Steps harborsteps.com, Western Ave. and University St.

Seattle Art Museum seattleartmuseum.org, 1300 1st Ave., 206-654-3100

Seattle Tower 1218 3rd Ave.

Rainier Square rainier-square.com, 4th Ave. and University St.

ACT Theatre acttheatre.org, 700 Union St., 206-292-7676

Freeway Park seattle.gov/parks, 700 Seneca St.

Plymouth Church Seattle plymouthchurchseattle.org, 1217 6th Ave., 206-622-4865

Seattle Central Library spl.org, 1000 4th Ave., 206-386-4636

Safeco Plaza safeco.com, 1001 4th Ave.

Colman Building 811 1st Ave.

ROUTE SUMMARY

1. Start at Western Ave. and University St. Climb the outdoor stairs, or take the elevator, to 1st Ave.

2. Cross 1st at University. Take the steps outside the Seattle Art Museum to 2nd Ave.

3. Cross kitty-corner at 2nd and University to the 1201 Third Avenue Building. Take the escalator to, then exit through, the 3rd Ave. lobby.

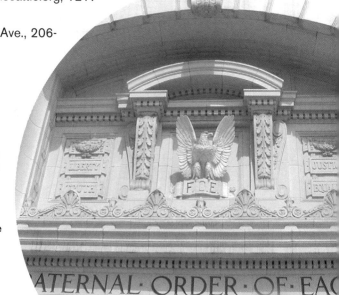

Eagles Auditorium

4. Cross 3rd and enter the Seattle Tower lobby. Take the elevators to the fifth floor. Take a right and leave through the skybridge to the Financial Center. Descend that building's plaza stairs.

5. Cross kitty-corner at 4th and University. Take the south entrance into Rainier Square; turn right at the signs for the pedestrian concourse. Take this passageway to its end.

6. Take the escalator up to Two Union Square's food court. Walk toward a small fireplace, then take a left and a right to another escalator. Take it up into the building's upper plaza level. Walk ahead to a pedestrian skybridge.

7. Take the path to the Convention Center's second floor.

8. Take the escalator or elevator to the fourth floor; exit the exterior doors to your east into Freeway Park.

9. Zigzag through Freeway Park to the outdoor plaza at 6th Ave. and Seneca St. Cross kitty-corner.

10. Go southeast on 6th one block.

11. Turn southwest on Spring St. to 5th Ave. and enter the Central Library. Take the escalator down and exit at 4th Ave.

12. Cross 4th Ave. at Madison St. Enter Safeco Plaza. Take the elevators or escalators down, then exit onto 3rd Ave.

13. Cross kitty-corner at 3rd and Madison. Walk through the Wells Fargo Center lobby; take an outdoor escalator to 2nd and Marion St.

14. Cross kitty-corner to the Exchange Building. Take its elevators to, and exit through, its 1st Ave. level.

15. Cross 1st at Marion. Walk on Marion back to Western, or take a skybridge to the ferry terminal.

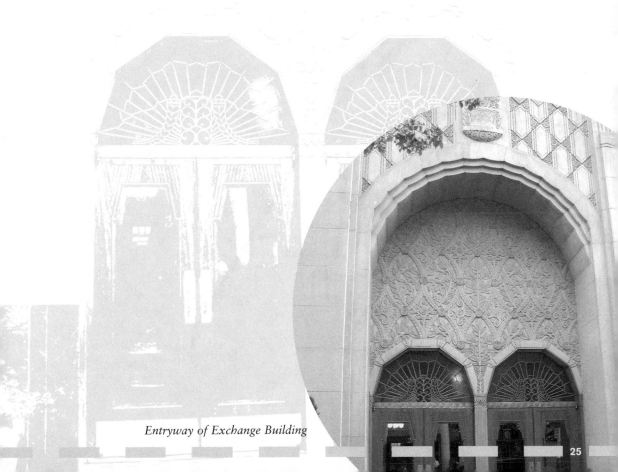

Entryway of Exchange Building

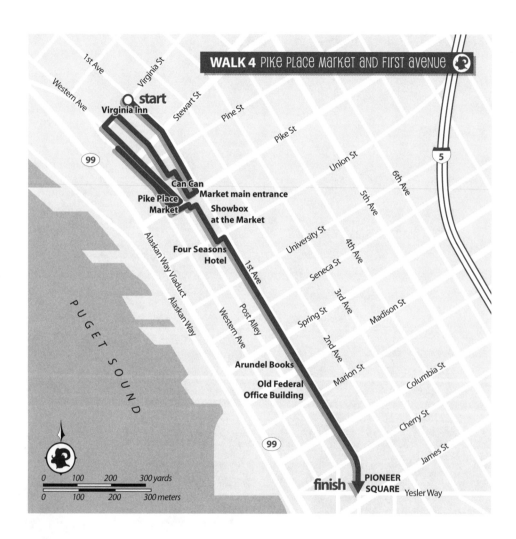

WALK 4 Pike Place Market and First Avenue

1st Ave
Virginia St
Western Ave
Stewart St
start
Virginia Inn
Pine St
Pike St
99
Union St
6th Ave
5th Ave
5
Can Can
Market main entrance
Pike Place
Market
Showbox
at the Market
4th Ave
Four Seasons
Hotel
University St
1st Ave
Seneca St
3rd Ave
Alaskan Way Viaduct
Spring St
Madison St
Alaskan Way
Post Alley
Western Ave
2nd Ave
P U G E T   S O U N D
Arundel Books
Marion St
Columbia St
Old Federal
Office Building
Cherry St
99
James St
0   100   200   300 yards
0   100   200   300 meters
finish
PIONEER
SQUARE
Yesler Way

4 Pike Place Market and First Avenue: Where Farmers Met Sailors

BOUNDARIES: **1st Ave., Virginia St., Yesler Way, and Western Ave.**
DISTANCE: **1½ miles**
DIFFICULTY: **Easy (all flat or downhill)**
PARKING: **Limited metered street parking; pay lots and garages include the Pike Place Market garage at Western and Pine St.**
PUBLIC TRANSIT: **Metro routes #15, 18, 21, 22, and 56 stop at 1st Ave. and Virginia St. The Transit Tunnel's Westlake Station has an exit at 3rd Ave. and Pine St.**

For more than 100 years, Pike Place has been home to the oldest continuously operating farmers' market in the United States. It's a fascinating concoction of produce, flowers, crafts, antiques, magic, and more. And it's a human-scale labyrinth of small buildings in assorted shapes and sizes, hugging a bluff looming over the waterfront. The Market abuts First Avenue, once a rowdy hangout for the waterfront's working men. Both districts have been spruced up but not fully bleached out. Hint: To get the most out of this walk, avoid the Market's peak tourist days (especially summer Saturdays).

● **Start at 1st Ave., heading southeast from Virginia St.** At this intersection's southeast corner, the 11-story Terminal Sales Building was built in 1923 as showrooms for manufacturers and wholesalers. Now it has high-ceilinged loft offices. Its ground-floor storefronts include the Peter Miller architectural bookstore. At its southwest corner, the century-old Virginia Inn bar and bistro denotes the start of the Pike Place Market Historic District.

Continue along 1st for three blocks, past colorful places to shop (including Metsker Maps and Dragon's Toy Box) and eat (Le Pichet, Bayou on First, and The Crumpet Shop). Just before Pike, take in the brassy animated sign for the Déjà Vu strip club, a remnant of 1st Ave.'s grittier former character. (*Déjà vu* is a French term that means, "Eh, nothin' ya haven't seen before.") Up Pike between 1st and 2nd is a big neon guitar above a Hard Rock Cafe. But the sign you're looking for is to your right on Pike. It's the historic PUBLIC MARKET CENTER sign with its proudly analog neon clock. Take a right into the market. Then immediately take another right into the Corner Market Building's lower arcade level, past the Can Can cabaret.

- Go northwest through the Corner Market and the adjacent Sanitary Public Market building, past ethnic food stands, a meat market, a dairy store, and more. At this corridor's northern end take a left to enter Post Alley, an outdoor promenade offering more snacking and shopping.

- Head northwest on Post Alley for three blocks. You find restaurants and bars of many types and price points (including the Irish-style Kell's and the Italian-style Pink Door), a tearoom, and a boutique hotel. You end up back at Virginia.

- Go southwest on Virginia to the northeast side of Pike Place. Stroll along the Market's main drag back to Pike St. Along your way are hundreds of tourists, depending on the season; plus Indian, Mexican, and Filippino groceries, sausage and humbow stands, the historic Three Girls bakery and sandwich counter, and what's billed as the world's first Starbucks Coffee store. (The real first Starbucks was in a now-razed building a block away.)

- When you get back to the L-shaped intersection of Pike Place and Pike St., hang a right. You're now facing the Market's Main Arcade, under the clock. Two of the Market's most-photographed attractions are here—Rachel the full-size piggy bank (proceeds from her coin slot benefit services for downtown seniors and low-income residents), and the Pike Place Fish Co. with its high-energy staffers tossing fish. Before you enter this section, look up to view five paintings by Aki Sogabe commemorating the Japanese-American farmers who sold produce here before they were sent to relocation camps during World War II.

- Walk northwest along the Main Arcade. Besides more tourists, you spot the Market's original raison d'etre, the "low stall" and "high stall" produce stands. (The former are farmer-run; the latter are year-round retail ventures.) You also see two popular-price restaurant bars with spectacular waterfront views (the Athenian and Lowell's), a closet-sized souvenir store, and another fish market (Pure Food Fish). The Main Arcade directly leads into the North Arcade, a long line of tables with artists and craftspeople.

- Turn around at the North Arcade's end. Backtrack past the craft sellers until you get back to the Main Arcade's northwesterly end. You see a ramp to the Down Under shops. Descend into a plank-floored indoor corridor of shops selling magic supplies, posters, postcards, beads, health food, candy, comic books, vintage clothing, and more.

- The southern end of the Down Under Arcade leads to exterior doors, which lead to the Pike Street Hillclimb, an elevator and series of outdoor stairs leading six stories from the Market's main level down to the waterfront. Take the stairs or elevator back to the south end of the Main Arcade. When you near Rachel the Pig, take a right-left dogleg into the Economy Market, a short series of stands and storefronts paralleling the end of Pike St. Its attractions include a magazine stand, a mini-donut stand, and an Italian deli and wine shop.

- Along the Economy Market's south wall, find a signed passageway leading to the Economy Market Atrium. Go through the atrium, a two-story indoor agora with shops selling western wear, wind-up toys, and herbal supplements. This room's southern end has a doorway marked TO MORE SHOPS AND RESTAURANTS. Take it into the indoor corridor of the South Arcade, a new building anchored by the Pike Pub and Brewery. It leads to 1st Ave. and Union St.

- Return to 1st. To your left, across the Showbox at the Market is a vintage big-band ballroom and one of Seattle's premiere music venues. Take a right across Union and walk southeast eight blocks along 1st. Where sailors and dockworkers once downed beers and watched pornos now stand galleries, bistros, a new Four Seasons Hotel, and an expanded Seattle Art Museum. (The

1st Avenue from Seattle Art Museum

latter occupies the lower levels of the Russell Investments Center, formerly WaMu Center, the second tower built by the now-deceased Washington Mutual Bank.)

At 1st and Spring, McCormick & Schmick's is a steak-and-seafood restaurant with a late-night bar menu. One block down at Madison, the Alexis Hotel houses both a real bookstore (Arundel Books) and a cafe and bar that looks like one (the Bookstore Bar & Cafe). Across Madison, the Old Federal Office Building is a brick-and-aluminum art deco treasure, a fine complement to the Colman Building one block away at Marion Street (Walk 3). At Cherry St., the 1903 Lowman Building has a French Renaissance–inspired gabled roof line. That building abuts Pioneer Square, which takes you one more block to Yesler Way.

CONNECTING THE WALKS

This walk connects easily to five other walks. It crosses Walk 3 at 1st and University. Its start crosses Walk 5. Its end crosses Walks 1 and 7. At 1st and Pine you're two blocks southwest of Walk 2.

POINTS OF INTEREST

Virginia Inn virginiainnseattle.com, 1937 1st Ave., 206-728-1937

Metsker Maps metskers.com, 1511 1st Ave., 206-623-8747

Pike Place Market pikeplacemarket.org, 1st Ave. and Pike St., 206-682-7453

Can Can thecancan.com, 94 Pike St., 206-652-0832

Showbox at the Market showboxonline.com, 1426 1st Ave., 206-628-3151

Four Seasons Hotel and Condos fourseasons.com/seattle, 99 Union St., 206-749-7000

Arundel Books arundelbookstores.com, 1001 1st Ave., 206-624-4442

route summary

1. Start at the southwest side of 1st Ave., south of Virginia St. Continue along 1st to Pike St.
2. Take a right into the market, then immediately take another right into the Corner Market.
3. Go northwest through the Corner Market and adjacent buildings, through to Post Alley.
4. Take Post Alley northwest for three blocks, back to Virginia.
5. Go southwest on Virginia to Pike Place itself. Stroll along Pike Place's east side back to Pike St. and the Main Arcade.
6. Walk northwest along the Main Arcade, which leads directly into the North Arcade.
7. Turn around at the North Arcade's end. Take the ramp down to the Down Under shops.
8. At the southern end of the Down Under arcade, climb the stairs back to the south end of the Main Arcade. Take a right-left dogleg into the Economy Market Atrium.
9. Go through the South Arcade building to 1st Ave. and Union St.
10. Return to 1st and walk southeast to Yesler Way.

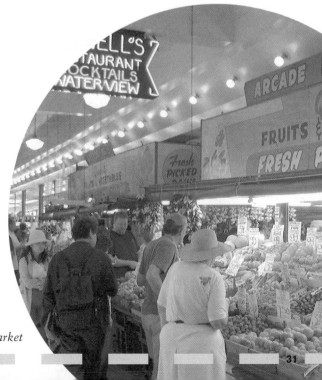

High stalls at the Pike Place Market

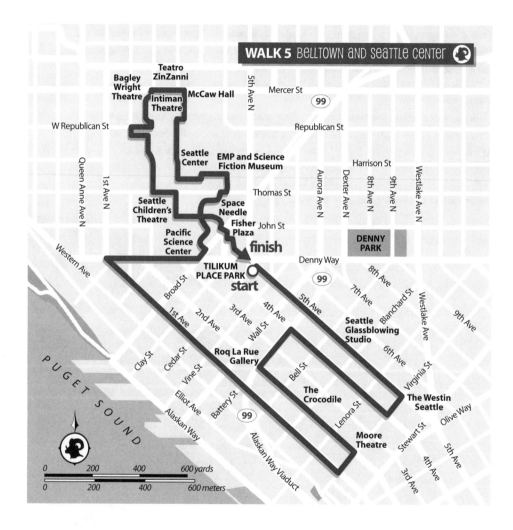

Teatro
ZinZanni

Bagley
Wright
Theatre

Intiman
Theatre

McCaw Hall

5th Ave N

Mercer St

99

W Republican St

Republican St

Queen Anne Ave N

1st Ave N

Seattle
Center

EMP and Science
Fiction Museum

Harrison St

Aurora Ave N

Dexter Ave N

8th Ave N

9th Ave N

Westlake Ave N

Thomas St

Seattle
Children's
Theatre

Space
Needle

Fisher
Plaza

John St

Pacific
Science
Center

finish

DENNY
PARK

Western Ave

TILIKUM
PLACE PARK

start

Denny Way

99

8th Ave

7th Ave

Blanchard St

Westlake Ave

9th Ave

Broad St

1st Ave

2nd Ave

3rd Ave

4th Ave

5th Ave

Seattle
Glassblowing
Studio

6th Ave

Virginia St

Clay St

Cedar St

Vine St

Roq La Rue
Gallery

Wall St

Bell St

The
Crocodile

Lenora St

The Westin
Seattle

Olive Way

Elliot Ave

Battery St

99

The
Crocodile

Moore
Theatre

Stewart St

5th Ave

4th Ave

3rd Ave

Alaskan Way

Alaskan Way Viaduct

PUGET SOUND

0   200   400   600 yards

0   200   400   600 meters

5 BELLTOWN AND SEATTLE CENTER: ALL YESTERDAY'S TOMORROWS

BOUNDARIES: **5th Ave., Virginia St., Warren Ave. N., and Mercer St.**
DISTANCE: **4 miles, in two segments**
DIFFICULTY: **Easy (all flat or slight inclines)**
PARKING: **Metered street parking; pay lots along Denny Way east of Broad St.**
PUBLIC TRANSIT: **Metro routes #3, 4, 8, 16, 19, 24, and 33 stop near this walk's start.**

In 1962, local civic leaders mounted the Century 21 Exposition, a world's fair celebrating what our world was supposed to have become by now. While we don't yet have domed cities or flying cars, we've kept the fair's grounds as a place for theater, opera, sports, science exhibits, and festivals. It all occurs under the watchful gaze and wasp-waisted stance of the Space Needle, one of the world's most recognizable icons. Seattle's prime symbol also looks over Belltown and the Denny Regrade, neighborhoods long overlooked by many. Where the fair's monorail once passed above car lots, printing plants, and nondescript commercial buildings, residential towers now scrape the sky and fashionable restaurants and boutiques beckon.

● **Start at Tilikum Place Park at the triangle of 5th Ave., Cedar St., and Denny Way. You're near what was the northern end of Denny Hill. The steep hill rose more than 100 feet, impeding the city's northern growth in the horse-and-wagon days. It was removed in three massive regrades from 1906 to 1929.**

Since 1912, cobblestoned Tilikum Place has been home to a statue of the city's namesake, Chief Seattle (also spelled "Sealth" and "Si'ahl" in the imprecise transliteration of his Lushootseed language). His arm is outstretched to welcome the first white settlers—not necessarily to lead them to the 5 Point Cafe (a lovingly preserved 24-hour dive diner and bar).

● **Turn southeast along 5th Ave. You're underneath the bulky concrete track of the Monorail, created to bring World's Fair visitors to the downtown core. At Wall St., the 1948 Post-Intelligencer building, a full-block slab of Truman-era concrete, is now gussied up for office tenants. On 5th's northeast side between Bell and Blanchard, a bizarre mural** advertises the "Wexley School for Girls." It's really an ad agency with a retro name and kitschy decor (rubber chickens hang inside its front windows). Across the street is the Seattle Glassblowing Studio, where you can buy decorative glass art and watch it being made.

Beyond 5th and Blanchard St., Top Pot Doughnuts occupies a stunning glass-fronted midcentury building. At Virginia St. looms the twin-cylindered Westin Hotel. The formerly Seattle-based chain has been at this location since 1928. The current towers were built in 1969 and 1982.

● Turn southwest along Virginia. Across from the Westin, the Icon Grill serves upscale comfort food under a ceiling crammed with Chihuly-style glass art. Behind it lies Escala, one of the most grandiose of our late-2000s condo megaprojects. Virginia and 4th is ground zero for celebrity restaurateur Tom Douglas, with his creations Lola, Dahlia Lounge, Dahlia Bakery, and Serious Pie. A neon caricature of Douglas holding a wriggling fish stands outside Dahlia. Sub Pop, the record label that turned "grunge" into a worldwide craze, has its offices in that building.

● Turn northwest along 4th. The 1963 Cinerama theater at Lenora St. is a

Back Story: The Regrade

Belltown's walkability results from Seattle's own *Extreme Makeover: City Edition*. Early city leaders decided that 100-foot-tall Denny Hill, just northwest of downtown, stood in the way of urban growth. Horse-drawn wagons could not carry merchandise over it. From 1902 to 1911, some 27 blocks were sluiced down flat. By the time it was done, the Ford Model T had made horse-drawn delivery obsolete. The rest of the hill, from Fifth to Westlake avenues, was steam-shoveled away from 1929 to 1930.

plain box on the outside, but a streamlined movie palace inside. On the same block is Yuki's Diffusion hair salon, run by Yuki Ohno. (You might have heard of his kid, skating champ Apolo Anton Ohno.) Beyond Bell St., the Two Bells Bar and Grill is a Repeal-era tavern serving art shows and thick burgers.

- Turn southwest at 4th and Battery. The handsome, brick-clad Fire Station #2 is the oldest in the city still operating. Kitty-corner from there, the black-glassed Fourth and Battery Building is Belltown's earliest "new" office tower (built in 1974). Two blocks away at 2nd Ave., Buckley's sports bar inhabits an art deco gem that had been MGM's regional office. This stretch of 2nd is Film Row, a onetime hotbed of distribution offices, film vaults, and theater-supply companies.

- Turn southeast along 2nd. City Hostel Seattle, next to Buckley's, was originally the William Tell Hotel, where studio sales reps (and at least a few movie stars) stayed while visiting Film Row. Across 2nd, Suyama Space is a big, rustic art space in the back of an architectural office. Next to that, the Rendezvous restaurant and lounge was originally a theater design and building company; its exquisite Jewel Box Theatre was that company's showroom. Next to that, RKO's old Film Row office is the Roq La Rue gallery, specializing in pop surrealism.

- At 2nd and Bell St., Mama's Mexican Kitchen has served Cal-Mex feasts and Elvis-dominated kitsch since 1974. It starts a block of hip drinking and music spots. The Crocodile, one of Seattle's top rock clubs for two decades, stands at the block's other end at 2nd and Blanchard. One block away at 2nd and Lenora, the facade of the 1914 Crystal Pool now clothes a condo tower's base.

  A block away at Virginia St., the Moore Theatre, a magnificent 1907 vaudeville palace, still hosts touring concerts and shows. Its ground-floor storefronts include the boutiques Fancy (jewelry and metal decorative pieces) and Schmancy (quirky toys and collectibles). Turn southwest along Virginia to 1st Ave. and the Terminal Sales Building (Walk 4).

- Turn northwest along 1st for 11 blocks to enjoy Seattle's prime see-and-be-seen nightlife scene. These joints range from loud DJ clubs to swank wine bars to quiet supper clubs to fashionably dark cocktail houses to boisterous meet-markets to smarty-arty hangouts to ex-dive bars gone legit. Many of these are open for daytime dining. This stretch of 1st Ave. also offers fashionable shopping, including stationery, clothes, and home furnishings.

And there's plenty of classic architecture among the newer condos—the Vogue Hotel (now the Vain hair salon), the 1889 Odd Fellows hall (now a pub), the 1889 Hull Building (now a fashion boutique), the Austin A. Bell Building (whose facade now stands in front of a condo structure), the Sailors Union of the Pacific (now a bar and restaurant), the Electrical Workers' hall (now a church), and the King County Labor Temple (still union offices!).

- Turn east along Denny Way's north side, and continue for five blocks, to Broad St. You pass Tini Bigs (a bar named for its "big [mar]tinis"), Champion Party Supply (a year-round Halloween party headquarters), and the new First United Methodist Church (a modern replacement for the building that's now Daniels Recital Hall, Walk 2).

- If you'd like to stop, continue along Denny back to 5th Ave. If you're continuing, turn northeast at Denny and Broad for less than a block, to Seattle Center's first pedestrian entrance.

- Meander north through this pathway, toward the Space Needle. Along the way you pass through *Olympic Iliad,* Alexander Liberman's sculpture made from orange metal tubes. You also pass a meditation garden donated by the Sri Chinmoy Foundation.

- Turn east at the Needle's north side, parallel to its main entrance. Even if you don't visit the 605-foot tower's restaurant or observation deck, you can admire the graceful curves of its tripod and UFO-esque "tophouse." Turn north in front of the west side of the Experience Music Project and Science Fiction Museum. Microsoft cofounder Paul Allen commissioned architect Paul Gehry's bold structure (designed without straight corners) as a tribute to rock music (and, some claim, to Allen's ego).

- From EMP's western entrance walk west, into the east entrance of Center House. The 1939 armory was one of several pre-fair buildings that were incorporated into the

Century 21 grounds. Take the stairs up to its main floor and food court, known during the fair as the Food Circus. Exit at Center House's west side.

- Head north past the International Fountain, a 1985 replacement for the fair's high-streaming centerpiece spectacle. Turn east at the Kobe Bell (a gift from Seattle's Japanese sister city) toward the elaborately lit courtyard of McCaw Hall. Home to Seattle Opera and Pacific Northwest Ballet, it's the third incarnation of the 1928 Civic Auditorium. Follow this courtyard out of the Center to Mercer St.

- Go west on Mercer. On the street's north side is Teatro ZinZanni, a circus-style dinner theater inside a high-tech "show tent." Reenter Seattle Center just west of 2nd Ave. N.

- This entrance leads you, heading south, toward the Bagley Wright Theatre (home of the Seattle Repertory Theatre). Pass this building's curvy, glassy front side. Then turn west to the Center's Warren Ave. N./Republican St. entrance. There's an open wooden doorway planted here, a memorial to renowned playwright August Wilson.

- Turn south and down a small flight of outdoor stairs, through a passage between the two Northwest Court buildings. These exhibit spaces are now home to the Vera Project, a teen-centric arts center. Turn east and then south beside KeyArena, created in 1995 with components from the fair-era Coliseum. It was built because the SuperSonics basketball team said they'd leave town without a new arena. Thirteen years later they left anyway. Continue south to Thomas St.

Space Needle at sunrise

- Head east along the back of Fisher Pavilion. Built into a hillside, its entire roof is an outdoor plaza.

- Turn south in front of Seattle Children's Theatre (also known as the Charlotte Martin Theatre), a handsome 1993 addition to a 1956 Shrine temple. You soon reach the main entrance to Pacific Science Center. Minoru Yamasaki (Walk 2) designed this sextet of clean white boxes with his trademark vertical trim features, surrounding reflecting pools, and streamlined, Gothic-inspired arches. Its recently-added IMAX Dome screens first-run 3D movies.

- Turn east, past the south side of the Mural Ampitheater, a performance space with Paul Horiuchi's 60-foot-long *Seattle Mural* as its backdrop. Continue east to the Space Needle's south side. Turn southeast through a circular plaza surrounding a fountain. Leave the Center at the triangular intersection of Broad St., John St., and 4th Ave. N.

- Cross Broad St. toward Fisher Plaza. Walk a southeasterly dogleg between its two buildings. At the northwest corner of 5th and Denny, you can see the Needle framed by KOMO-TV's satellite dishes on Fisher Plaza's roof. Before you cross Denny back to Tilikum Place, look east for the pink neon sign announcing the Elephant Super Car Wash.

CONNECTING THE WALKS

This walk connects easily to four other walks. At 4th and Virginia you're two blocks northwest of Walk 2. At 1st and Virginia you're at the start of Walk 4. This walk's 1st Ave. stretch is three blocks east of Walk 7. At Warren and Republican you're one block east of Walk 8.

POINTS OF INTEREST

5 Point Cafe the5pointcafe.com, 415 Cedar St., 206-448-9993

Seattle Glassblowing Studio seattleglassblowing.com, 2227 5th Ave., 206-448-2181

Westin Seattle starwoodhotels.com/westin/seattle, 1900 5th Ave., 206-728-1000

The Crocodile thecrocodile.com, 2200 2nd Ave., 206-441-7416

Moore Theatre stgpresents.org, 1932 2nd Ave., 206-443-1744

Seattle Center seattlecenter.com, 305 Harrison St., 206-684-7200

Space Needle spaceneedle.com, 400 Broad St., 206-905-2100

Experience Music Project and Science Fiction Museum empsfm.org, 325 5th Ave. N., 877-EMP-SFM1

Teatro ZinZanni zinzanni.org, 222 Mercer St., 206-802-0015

Pacific Science Center pacsci.org, 200 2nd Ave. N., 206-443-2001

route summary

1. Start at Tilikum Place Park at the triangle of 5th Ave., Cedar St., and Denny Way.

2. Turn southeast along 5th Ave., and continue for seven blocks, to Virginia St.

3. Turn southwest along Virginia, and continue for one block, to 4th Ave.

4. Turn northwest along 4th, and continue for four blocks, to Battery St.

5. Turn southwest along Battery, and continue for two blocks, to 2nd Ave.

6. Turn southeast along 2nd, and continue for five blocks, to Virginia St.

7. Turn southwest along Virginia, and continue for one block, to 1st Ave.

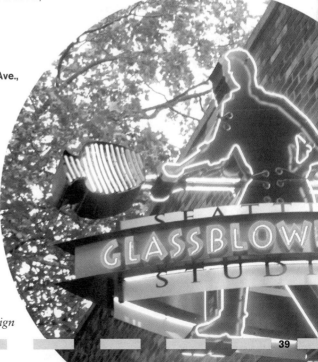

Seattle Glassblowing Studio sign

8.   Turn northwest along 1st, and continue for 12 blocks, to Denny Way.

9.   Turn east along Denny, and continue for five blocks, to Broad St.

10. Turn northeast along Broad. Walk for less than a block, to Seattle Center's first pedestrian entrance.

11. Go north through this path toward the Space Needle. Turn east at the Needle's north side.

12. Turn north in front of the west side of the Experience Music Project and Science Fiction Museum.

13. From EMP's west side walk west, into Center House. Take the stairs up to its main floor; leave at its west side.

14. Head north, past the International Fountain, through the courtyard in front of McCaw Hall and out to Mercer St.

15. Go west on Mercer a little more than one block, to just west of 2nd Ave. N.

16. Reenter the center grounds. Walk past the Bagley Wright Theatre's front; then turn west to the August Wilson memorial at the Center's Warren Ave. N./Republican St. entrance.

17. Turn south through the Northwest Court buildings. Turn east and then south alongside KeyArena. Continue south to Thomas St.

18. Head east, alongside the upper plaza of Fisher Pavilion.

19. Turn south in front of Seattle Children's Theatre, to the Pacific Science Center's main entrance.

20. Walk east from here, to the Space Needle's south side.

21. Turn southeast; leave the Center grounds at the intersection of Broad St., John St., and 4th Ave. N.

22. Cross Broad. Walk southeast between the two buildings of Fisher Plaza, back to 5th and Denny.

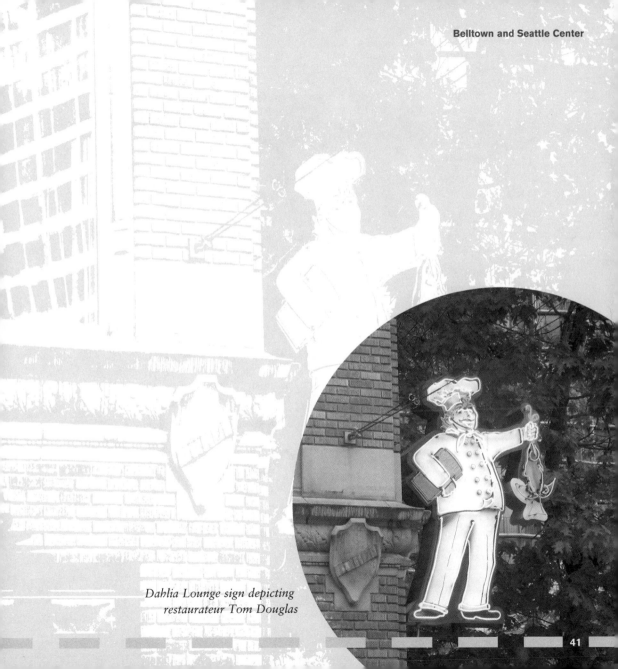

*Dahlia Lounge sign depicting
restaurateur Tom Douglas*

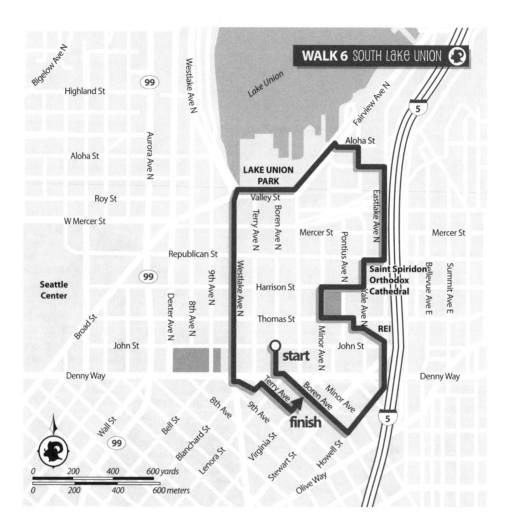

Bigelow Ave N

99

Highland St

Westlake Ave N

Lake Union

Fairview Ave N

5

Aloha St

Aloha St

Aurora Ave N

LAKE UNION PARK

Roy St

Valley St

Terry Ave N

Boren Ave N

W Mercer St

Mercer St

Eastlake Ave N

Mercer St

Republican St

Pontius Ave N

99

Saint Spiridon Orthodox Cathedral

Bellevue Ave E

Summit Ave E

Seattle Center

Dexter Ave N

8th Ave N

9th Ave N

Westlake Ave N

Harrison St

Yale Ave N

REI

Broad St

Thomas St

John St

Minor Ave N

John St

start

Denny Way

Terry Ave

Boren Ave

Minor Ave

Denny Way

8th Ave

9th Ave

finish

5

Wall St

Bell St

Blanchard St

Lenora St

Virginia St

Stewart St

Howell St

99

Olive Way

0   200   400   600 yards
0   200   400   600 meters

6 SOUTH LAKE UNION: (PAUL) ALLEN-TOWN

BOUNDARIES: **Boren Ave. N., Eastlake Ave. N., Fairview Ave. N., Valley St., and Westlake Ave. N.**
DISTANCE: **2¾ miles**
DIFFICULTY: **Moderate (two brief uphill segments, one toward the end)**
PARKING: **Metered street parking; pay lots and garages include a lot at Boren Ave. and Lenora St.**
PUBLIC TRANSIT: **The Seattle Streetcar stops at 9th Ave., Westlake Ave., and Blanchard St. Metro routes #8 and 70 stop along Fairview Ave. N.**

This former low-rent district northeast of downtown has blossomed, thanks in part to Microsoft cofounder Paul Allen's many real estate ventures. Many big and shiny office, residential, and retail projects have turned much of south Lake Union into a high-tech fantasy land, complete with its own neighborhood trolley. That's not to say there was nothing there before. For decades, city officials vowed to maintain Lake Union as a "working lake," and the blocks south of the lake still hold onto a lot of industry, history, and a particular rustic beauty. It's a place where one of the original "grunge" music clubs, an ornate little orthodox church, and a mammoth nonprofit outdoors store coexist in mutual tolerance.

● Start outside the 13 Coins restaurant at Boren Ave. N. and John St. Since 1967, this 24-hour diner and steakhouse has defined affordable class, and has been a hangout for employees of the *Seattle Times*. The paper's 1930 Moderne headquarters stands across Boren on John, along with several annex buildings added while newsprint was a thriving industry.

● Walk south to Boren and Denny Way. Dogleg east on Denny and back onto Boren, walking southeast. You soon find the gently sloped wood structure that's now Cornish College of the Arts' Raisbeck Performance Hall. The 1915 timbered structure was originally a Sons of Norway Hall; later it housed a series of gay dance clubs. A block and a half away at Boren and Stewart St., a nondescript, two-story Boilermakers' Union hall conceals the lavish yet comfy Washington Dance Club upstairs.

● Turn northeast at Boren and Howell St. On Howell's south side, the older of Martin Selig's two Metropolitan Park office buildings is known as the "Can of Spam

Building." Across from it is Re-bar, for two decades a straight and gay crossover DJ club and performance space. (It's where columnist Dan Savage once directed drag productions of female-lead stage plays.) The building also houses the Market House Deli, selling the best corned beef in town.

● Continue as Howell bends north into Eastlake Ave. Just beyond the Denny Way overpass is a long, gritty structure that's been a live music venue for more than four decades. It's now El Corazón, but it was the Off Ramp when all the pre-stardom grunge bands played there.

● Across Eastlake and John St. is the massive retail theater spectacle that is the flagship REI (Recreational Equipment Inc.) store. The sporting goods giant began as a cooperative buying service, outfitting serious mountain climbers. It's got a big climbing wall and an outdoor trail network (for test-riding mountain bikes and hiking shoes).

● Cross the south side of the REI complex, to Yale Ave. north of John. Cross Yale to Alley24, a full-block residential, retail, and office complex incorporating the brick facade of an old laundry building. It includes Snowboard Connection, a store that moved here from Pioneer Square to be near REI, and Lunchbox Laboratory, a gourmet burger emporium that moved here from Ballard to be near the office crowd.

● Exit Alley24 at its north side. Turn west on Thomas St. Beyond the intersection with Pontius Ave. N. (nobody's opened a Pilates studio on that street yet), the Cascade Playground and P-Patch combines green space with a community garden and a meeting hall. On the south side of Thomas, enjoy the century-old Immanuel Lutheran Church, a solid bulk of white-painted wood construction. On the northwest corner of Thomas and Minor Ave., Paddy Coynes is a "traditional Irish pub" at the bottom of a 2004 condo building.

● Turn north on Minor, and continue one block to Harrison St., in view of the P-Patch and its adjacent Garden of Happiness. Turn east on Harrison two blocks to Yale Ave. and St. Spiridon Orthodox Cathedral. This exquisite 1937 brick building was designed in the Russian church–style. It's even more stunning inside; the sanctuary is a tiny gem of art and iconography.

- Turn north on Yale, and continue one block to Republican St., past a new building with a German pub at its ground floor. Dogleg east on Republican one block back to Eastlake. (This block's a steep climb, but just for 200 feet.) At this intersection's southwest corner are two live-music bars, the Lo-Fi and Victory Lounge.

- Walk north on the west side of Eastlake, parallel to Interstate 5. North of Mercer St. is a classic brick apartment block containing sandwich place and music hotspot Cafe Venus and the Mars Bar. Continue on Eastlake on an overpass above the I-5 Mercer exit (the "Mercer Mess" to generations of frustrated commuters), to Aloha St. You're in "cancer country," the adjoining campuses of the Fred Hutchinson Cancer Research Center and the Seattle Cancer Care Alliance.

- Turn west on Aloha, and continue one block to Yale Ave. Turn north and walk one block to the traffic circle in front of the "Hutch" campus to see *Vessel*, artist Ed Carpenter's four-story sculpture made with colorful light tubes reaching toward the sky. Turn west from the traffic circle onto Ward St. heading westbound, and go one block to Fairview Ave. N. Cross Fairview, to the pedestrian and bicycle path on its northwest side.

- Turn southwest on Fairview, near the lake. You can see yacht docks from a distance here; if you want to see them up-close, turn into the Chandler's Cove Marina complex. It includes a small private park, shops, and restaurants. Shortly beyond, the Fairview path bends east, becoming parallel with Valley St. Look southeast at Valley and Fairview to see a stoic five-story brick building. It was originally a Ford Model T assembly plant; it later housed magazine printing presses, and is now rental storage units.

- Continue on the path north of Valley past Daniel's Broiler (a water-view steakhouse) and the Center for Wooden Boats and Northwest Seaport (two nonprofits preserving Seattle's seagoing heritage). See the new Lake Union Park, a vast open space hugging the lakeshore. The park's centerpiece is an old National Guard armory that will be the Museum of History and Industry's new home (Walk 20).

- Along this path north of Terry and west of Boren is a stop for the Seattle Streetcar, a 1.3-mile high-tech trolley installed at Paul Allen's urging. Some give it the unofficial nickname "South Lake Union Trolley," usually referred to by its acronym. Take the trolley west and then south on Westlake Ave., to Denny Way. Or walk this eight-block segment. If you walk it, you'll get to peek inside Antique Liquidators (a two-story warehouse of funky old things for sale), as well as view many shiny new projects built for Allen and other developers.

● On the east side of Westlake south of Denny, a new complex contains a Whole Foods Market and a Pan Pacific Hotel. Climb the steps or take the elevator here, to Terry Ave. Across Terry is the hulking, tall warehouse building that's now Cornish College's main campus. Founded by Nellie Cornish in 1914 as a music academy, it now teaches visual and performing arts, interior and graphic design, and video production.

● Turn southeast on Terry (a slight incline) to Virginia St.; follow Virginia back to Fairview.

CONNECTING THE WALKS

This walk connects easily to three other walks. Its midpoint at Fairview and Ward is near the start of Walk 22. It ends five blocks from Walk 2 and six blocks from Walk 5.

POINTS OF INTEREST

13 Coins 13coins.com, 125 Boren Ave. N., 206-682-2513

Raisbeck Performance Hall cornish.edu, 2015 Boren Ave., 206-726-5066

Re-bar rebarseattle.com, 1114 Howell St., 206-223-9873

El Corazón elcorazonseattle.com, 109 Eastlake Ave. E., 206-381-3094

REI rei.com/stores, 222 Yale Ave. N., 206-223-1944

Immanuel Lutheran Church immanuelseattle.org, 1215 Thomas St., 206-622-1930

St. Spiridon Orthodox Cathedral saintspiridon.org, 400 Yale Ave. N., 206-624-5341

Chandler's Cove Marina 901 Fairview Ave. N., 206-382-0090

Center for Wooden Boats cwb.org, 1010 Valley St., 206-382-2628

Cornish College of the Arts cornish.edu, 1000 Lenora St., 206-726-5151

route summary

1. Start at Boren Ave. N., walking south from John St. to Denny Way.

2. Dogleg east on Denny and back to Boren; resume walking southeast.

3. Turn northeast on Howell St., which bends north into Eastlake Ave.

4. Cross Eastlake at John St.

5. Walk across the south side of the REI complex, to Yale Ave. and John.

6. Cross Yale, to the Alley24 complex. Exit Alley 24 at its north side.

7. Turn west on Thomas St.

8. Turn north on Minor Ave.

9. Turn east on Harrison St.

10. Turn north on Yale Ave.

11. Dogleg east on Republican St. one block.

12. Turn north on Eastlake.

13. Turn west on Aloha St.

14. Dogleg north on Yale Ave. to the traffic circle.

15. Turn west on Ward St.

16. Turn southwest on Fairview Ave. N., which bends west into Valley St.

17. Walk (or take the Seattle Streetcar) south on Westlake Ave. N.

18. Climb the steps or take the elevator at 9th Ave. and Westlake.

19. Turn southeast on Terry Ave. to Virginia St.

20. Follow Virginia back to Fairview.

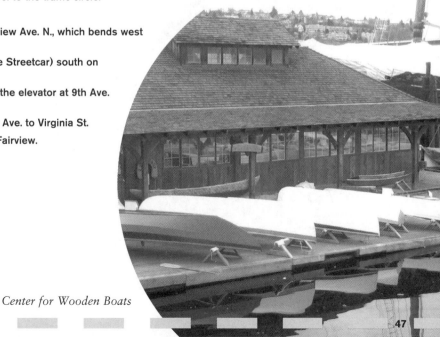

Center for Wooden Boats

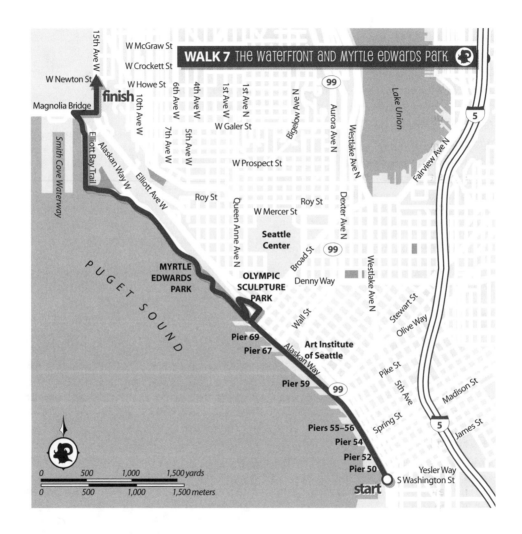

WALK 7 THE WATERFRONT AND MYRTLE EDWARDS PARK

15th Ave W

W McGraw St
W Crockett St
W Newton St
W Howe St

finish

Magnolia Bridge

W Galer St

99

10th Ave W
6th Ave W
4th Ave W
7th Ave W
5th Ave W

1st Ave N

Bigelow Ave N

Aurora Ave N

Lake Union

Westlake Ave N

Fairview Ave N

5

W Prospect St

Roy St

W Mercer St

Roy St

Dexter Ave N

Smith Cove Waterway

Elliott Bay Trail

Alaskan Way W

Elliott Ave W

Queen Anne Ave N

**Seattle
Center**

Broad St

99

**MYRTLE
EDWARDS
PARK**

**OLYMPIC
SCULPTURE
PARK**

Denny Way

Westlake Ave N

P U G E T   S O U N D

Wall St

Stewart St

Olive Way

Pier 69
Pier 67

Alaskan Way

**Art Institute
of Seattle**

Pier 59

99

Pike St

5th Ave

Madison St

Piers 55–56
Pier 54
Pier 52
Pier 50

Spring St

5

James St

Yesler Way
S Washington St

start

0   500   1,000   1,500 yards

0   500   1,000   1,500 meters

7 The Waterfront and Myrtle Edwards Park: Pier review

BOUNDARIES: Alaskan Way, S. Washington St., 15th Ave. W., and W. Howe St.
DISTANCE: 4 miles, in two segments
DIFFICULTY: Moderate (one short incline)
PARKING: Limited metered street parking; pay lots and garages include the Commuter Centre Garage, 809 Western Ave.
PUBLIC TRANSIT: Metro routes #15, 18, 21, 22, 56, and 57 stop at 1st Ave. and Yesler Way. Route #99 stops at Alaskan Way and S. Main St.

Seattle's blessed with big and small lakes and rivers and creeks and artificial cuts galore. But when Seattleites talk about "The Waterfront," they mean the central harbor on Elliott Bay. This city is here because its founders wanted to create a thriving seaport. It became a power-house with the aid of the Alaska and Asia/Pacific trade. When the freight moved to container docks to the south, the central waterfront's vintage docks and freight sheds got reinvented for tourism, recreation, and pleasure travel. In the 1970s, a mile and a half of Elliott Bay front-age became Myrtle Edwards Park, a strip of greenery abutting the blue bay. More recently, expanding it into Olympic Sculpture Park gave the area a collective front lawn.

● Start at the Public Boat Landing, Alaskan Way and S. Washington St. This ornate wrought-iron pergola is the perfect gateway from Pioneer Square (rock-solid yet frilly) to the Waterfront (all wood, creosote, and water). To the east, gaze at the 1950s concrete brutalism of the Alaskan Way Viaduct while you can. Politicians are itching to replace the elevated highway, once they agree on what to replace it with.

In getting here, you've probably crossed the Waterfront Streetcar tracks. From 1982 to 2005, refurbished 1930s trolleys from Melbourne, Australia, rolled along Alaskan Way, through Pioneer Square, and to the International District. They were mothballed when their garage was razed as part of the Olympic Sculpture Park. The line might not return until the Viaduct replacement project is done. For now, the free #99 bus covers its route.

- Walk northwest along the west side of Alaskan Way. Originally a wooden rail trestle over the water, it got filled in and paved in the early 20th century. Here's what you'll find, pier by pier (don't worry about numbers jumping ahead; some piers were razed or consolidated):

- Pier 50: The King County Water Taxi runs a passenger ferry service to Alki (Walk 33).

- Pier 52: The main Washington State Ferry Terminal, with car and passenger service to Bremerton and Bainbridge Island, is part of the world's third-largest ferry network. (Across from here are a sizeable antique mall and a youth clothing store.)

- Pier 53: Fire Station #5 is home of the city's fireboat fleet.

- Pier 54: This first of five classic wood-shed piers hosts Ivar's Acres of Clams, the Waterfront's anchor restaurant since 1938, when local radio personality Ivar Haglund started a private aquarium and roadside fish stand. It now offers indoor dining, plus an outdoor "fish bar" with bench seating under heat lamps. Also on Pier 54 is Ye Olde Curiosity Shop, a gift and novelty store (and home to a glass-encased mummy named Sylvester).

- Pier 55: Red Robin, the formerly Seattle-based burger chain, has a branch here. Outside, Argosy Cruises' nine boats offer sightseeing, dining, and party cruises around the Sound.

- Pier 56: Another Argosy dock abuts Elliott's Oyster House.

- Pier 57: A small amusement arcade (featuring a wooden carousel) lies behind a restaurant and an import shop.

- Pier 58: Waterfront Park is a concrete open space, seldom used for anything these days. (Across from here are the Highway 99 Blues Club and the Seattle Antiques Market.)

- Pier 59: The Seattle Aquarium features both local and exotic sea critters in 400,000 gallons of water. Across, at Alaskan and Pike, is the Pike Street Hillclimb, a public staircase and elevator up to the Pike Place Market (Walk 4) and downtown. You can take the Hillclimb, or continue on Alaskan.

- Piers 62–63: This wood-planked open space used to host summer concerts. Across Alaskan, condos and a hotel squeeze into a narrow strip of land between Alaskan, the Viaduct, and the railroad tracks.

- Piers 64–66: Three old wooden-shed piers were replaced in the 1990s by the Bell Street Pier complex. It includes a small-boat marina, a seafood restaurant, a now-closed maritime museum, a conference center, a cruise-ship terminal, and a pedestrian skybridge to Belltown (Walk 5). Across Alaskan stands part of the Art Institute of Seattle.

- Pier 67: The Edgewater Hotel is Seattle's only on-the-water hostelry. Once *the* local place for touring rock bands (and their female admirers, as noted in the Frank Zappa song "Mudshark") to stay, it's now gussied up with ski-lodge trappings and a water-view restaurant.

- Pier 69: The Victoria Clipper's day trips to Victoria, B.C. (and seasonally to other places, such as the La Conner tulip festival), depart here. Across Alaskan, a former can factory is now headquarters for the RealNetworks software firm.

- Pier 70: A 1902 fish-packing warehouse became a mini-mall and disco in 1972. In 1998 it was the main setting for MTV's series *The Real World*. It now houses law offices and an upscale restaurant. Across Alaskan, the Old Spaghetti Factory has served family meals since 1970 in a brick warehouse.

- At Pier 70, Alaskan Way turns into the northeast-heading Broad Street. Take Broad two uphill blocks to Western Ave. and the Olympic Sculpture Park's main entrance. The privately funded outdoor exhibit space (on the former Union 76 petroleum storage depot) is a nine-acre blend of lawns, trails, gardens, an indoor nature exhibit, and more than a dozen medium-to-huge, abstract-to-postmodern metal monuments.

- Take the Sculpture Park's 2,200-foot main path as it zigzags back to the waterfront, at the southern end of Myrtle Edwards Park. This walk's first segment ends here. You can take a #99 bus at Alaskan and Broad back to your start, or continue with segment two.

- Still with us? Then walk into Myrtle Edwards Park and follow its main trail heading northwest. This trail hugs the shoreline for 1.2 miles, starting with a short artificial beach (part of the Sculpture Park). From there it's paved trails, rocky shore, grass, and trees (and fenced-off freight tracks to your right).

Sights along your way through the park include the P-I Globe (a 30-foot steel-and-neon sign that advertised the sadly missed *Post-Intelligencer* newspaper, and still promotes its spinoff website), a small lighthouse statue (memorializing fishermen who died at sea), a rose garden, a fishing pier, and the Amgen Bridge (a pedestrian bridge with double-helix design features, leading to a biotech corporate campus). At one point, the path goes under a conveyor crane to a grain terminal.

● At the park's northern end, the trail bends north as the Terminal 91 Bike Path, maintained by the Port of Seattle. It parallels the Smith Cove Waterway, one of the Pacific Coast's largest vehicle import terminals. If you're lucky, you can spot Japan's latest models being driven off of freighter ships. Take this trail up to the Magnolia Bridge.

● Follow the signs onto the Magnolia Bridge's pedestrian lane and head east over the railroad tracks, to 15th Ave. W. and W. Garfield St. There's a neon-sign refurbishing yard here, with several quaint old signs lying around (some even plugged in and lit).

● Turn north and walk two blocks to a strip mall at 15th and W. Newton St., or take a #15 or 18 bus at 15th and Garfield back to Pioneer Square.

CONNECTING THE WALKS

This walk connects easily to a half dozen other walks. It starts two blocks from Walks 1 and 4. At Pier 50, you're at the start of Walk 33. At Alaskan and University you're one block southwest of Walk 3. At Western and Broad you're one block southwest of Walk 5 and seven blocks south of Walk 8.

POINTS OF INTEREST

King County Water Taxi kingcountyferries.org, Alaskan Way and Yesler Way, Pier 50, 206-684-1511

Washington State Ferry Terminal wsdot.wa.gov/ferries, 801 Alaskan Way, Pier 52, 206-464-6400

Ivar's Acres of Clams ivars.com, 1001 Alaskan Way, Pier 54, 206-624-6852

Argosy Cruises argosycruises.com, 1101 Alaskan Way, Piers 55–56, 206-642-7816

Seattle Aquarium seattleaquarium.org, 1483 Alaskan Way, Pier 59, 206-386-4320

Bell Street Pier portseattle.org, 2203 Alaskan Way, Pier 66, 206-615-3952

Edgewater Hotel edgewaterhotel.com, 2411 Alaskan Way, Pier 67, 206-728-7000

Victoria Clipper clippervacations.com, 2701 Alaskan Way, Pier 69, 206-888-2535

Olympic Sculpture Park seattleartmuseum.org, 2901 Western Ave., 206-654-3100

Myrtle Edwards Park seattle.gov/parks, 3130 Alaskan Way W., 206-684-4075

route summary

1. Start at the Public Boat Landing, Alaskan Way and S. Washington St.

2. Walk northwest along the west side of Alaskan Way.

3. Turn northeast on Broad St. to Western Ave.

4. Take the Olympic Sculpture Park's main path back to the waterfront.

5. Follow the main Myrtle Edwards Park trail to the Smith Cove Waterway.

6. Turn north onto the Terminal 91 Bike Path to the Magnolia Bridge.

7. Go east on the bridge, to 15th Ave. W. and W. Garfield St.

8. Turn north and walk two blocks to 15th and W. Newton St., or take a #15 or 18 bus at 15th and Garfield to near this walk's start.

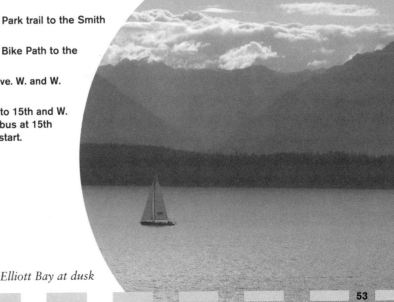

Elliott Bay at dusk

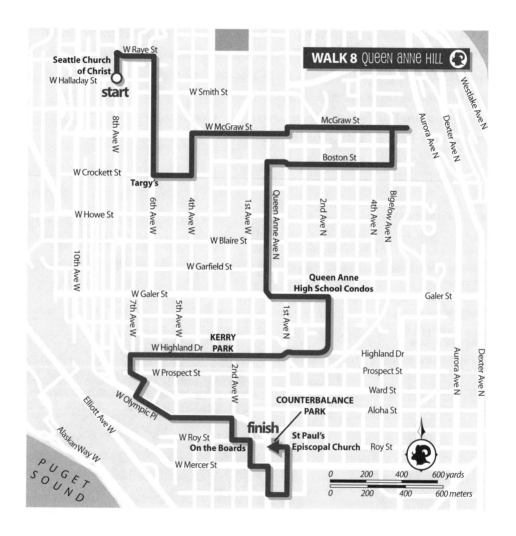

W Raye St

Seattle Church
of Christ
W Halladay St
start

W Smith St

8th Ave W

W McGraw St

W Crockett St

Targy's

6th Ave W

4th Ave W

W Howe St

W Blaire St

1st Ave W

W Garfield St

McGraw St

Boston St

Queen Anne Ave N

2nd Ave N

4th Ave N

Bigelow Ave N

Aurora Ave N

Dexter Ave N

Westlake Ave N

10th Ave W

W Galer St

7th Ave W

5th Ave W

1st Ave N

Queen Anne
High School Condos

Galer St

**KERRY
PARK**

W Highland Dr

W Prospect St

2nd Ave W

Highland Dr

Prospect St

Ward St

Aurora Ave N

Dexter Ave N

Elliott Ave W

W Olympic Pl

**COUNTERBALANCE
PARK**

Aloha St

finish

W Roy St

On the Boards

St Paul's
Episcopal Church

Roy St

AlaskanWay W

W Mercer St

P U G E T
S O U N D

| 0 | 200 | 400 | 600 yards |
| 0 | 200 | 400 | 600 meters |

8 QUEEN ANNE HILL: TOP OF THE TOWN

BOUNDARIES: 8th Ave. W., W. Raye St., Bigelow Ave. N., and Republican St.
DISTANCE: 4½ miles
DIFFICULTY: Moderate (one brief uphill segment)
PARKING: Free street parking
PUBLIC TRANSIT: Metro route #2 stops at 7th Ave. W. and W. Raye St.

Rising some 450 feet, Queen Anne is the tallest of Seattle's original "seven hills." Its name came from the ornate Victorian homes on its south slope, built to take advantage of some truly spectacular views. Atop the hill's view-deprived mesa, the housing stock tended to be more modest but still solid and respectable. This venerable middle-class neighborhood was becoming more regal even before the 2000s housing inflation. Today, you'll see an enticing mix of classic 20th-century homes, schools, and commercial architecture, as you walk down lovely tree-lined streets and catch stunning views of the city and Puget Sound.

- Start at 8th Ave. W. and W. Halladay St., outside the Seattle Church of Christ. The exquisite 1926 octagon combines Spanish colonial and Byzantine influences. It's the first of several former Christian Science buildings on these walks. Walk north on 8th one block.

- Turn right on W. Raye St. past Mount Pleasant Cemetery. Among those interred here are Seattle cofounders William and Sarah Bell (Walk 5), Children's Hospital cofounder Anna Herr Clise, and some of the ashes of labor organizer Joe Hill. It also has Jewish, Muslim, and Chinese burial areas.

- Turn south on 6th Ave. W. The vast majority of Seattle's 84 square miles are zoned as single-family neighborhoods. This typical street has low-rise houses, often Craftsman bungalows or similar styles, with well-groomed front yards and setback side lawns between each home. South of W. Smith St., Coe Elementary School is a 2003 structure resembling one that burned two years before. At W. McGraw St., Ken's Market could be described as either a huge deli-mart or tiny supermarket. At W. Crockett St., the stone-clad Targy's is an unapologetic working-stiffs' tavern.

- Turn east on Crockett to 4th Ave. W., another pleasant street with trees and shrubbery. Go north one block. Turn east on W. McGraw St., past the start of the Queen Anne business strip (which we'll cut back to).

- At 1st Ave. N. (which, in Seattle's idiosyncratic street nomenclature, is two blocks east of 1st Ave. W.), take a left-right dogleg back onto McGraw. Beyond 2nd Ave. N., McGraw becomes a short bridge over a deep wooded ravine. Continue to the street-end viewpoint east of Bigelow Ave. N., featuring a stunning vista of Lake Union and Capitol Hill.

- Backtrack to Bigelow and turn south. This is part of the "Crown of Queen Anne," a scenic loop encircling the hill. At Boston St., notice the sweeping brick solidity of the Old Hay School. (The school district built a new Hay Elementary a few blocks away, then kept the old Hay as an alternative secondary school.) You might glimpse the Space Needle to the south.

- Turn west on Boston. West of 3rd Ave. N., five attached skinny houses typify local townhome projects of the 2000s. A different townhome group at Warren Ave. N. makes four small homes look like one big one. Kitty-corner from there, a retirement home occupies the original 1908 and 1928 brick buildings of Seattle Children's Hospital (now in the Laurelhurst neighborhood).

- Turn south on Queen Anne Ave. N. The neighborhood's main drag is also called the "Counterbalance," from the gravity-assisted cable car that used to connect it with downtown. The street's gathered fashionable shops and restaurants, but also remains a place for basic provisions.

- East of Queen Anne Ave. at Galer St. is a pedestrian staircase. Climb it to 1st Ave. W. and Galer, and continue east. To your left, you see the new John Hay Elementary School (mentioned above). To your right, the KOMO-TV transmitting tower stands just before the former Queen Anne High School (now condos). The 1909 neoclassical building typifies Progressive-era desires to edify as well as educate.

- Turn south on 2nd Ave. N., a narrow street with thick trees. It bends west into Highland Drive. At Highland and 1st Ave. N., the 1906 Polson mansion combines Arts and Crafts architecture with a turreted round tower on its view side. Across 1st N. is the Chappel House, built in a French Gothic motif.

As the views get better, the houses get ritzier. At the southwest corner of Queen Anne and Highland is the 1905 Harry W. Treat House. The 17,000-square-foot brick-and-stucco mansion is now divided into 15 apartments. Across the street, the white colonial Ballard mansion is also now apartments. The buildings built *as* apartments get fancier too; particularly the 1921 Victoria Apartments (now condos), a block-long, four-story brick estate with a meticulous front garden.

The next block up is Kerry Park, whose downtown-skyline vista is familiar to every *Frasier* viewer. Continue west on Highland, enjoying the variety of street trees and the stately Victorian and Queen Anne homes. The Betty Bowen Viewpoint, named for a local arts patron, lies at 7th Ave. W. Besides a stunning view toward Elliott Bay and the Pier 86 grain terminals (Walk 7), it has sidewalk mosaics representing Pacific Northwest artists.

● Turn south on 7th, a narrow cobblestone road. Take an east dogleg turn onto W. Prospect St., then promptly go southeast on W. Kinnear Pl. To your left at 700 W. Kinnear, what was a large, tasteful 1900 home was recently enlarged and altered into an ostentatious monument to excess. You can see what it used to look like on an episode of HBO's *Six Feet Under*.

● Turn southwest back onto 7th (another steep downhill brick road) to W. Olympic Pl. At the northeast corner are the Chelsea Apartments, a 1907 English Renaissance hotel building. Across Olympic lies Kinnear Park, with another lookout toward Elliott Bay (restrooms are in a dugout structure beneath the lookout).

● Turn southeast on Olympic, which soon bends east. At Olympic and 5th Ave. W., a new row of faux-Tudor townhomes tries to fit in alongside older, Spanish mission–style apartments. At 2nd Ave. W., the 1909 De La Mar Apartments are four stories of neoclassical stateliness with marble floors and stained-glass windows. You are forgiven if you mistake the building for a European embassy.

● Turn south on 2nd, and continue past several modest prewar apartment low-rises. Turn east onto W. Roy St., to an old brick church that's now On the Boards, home to contemporary dance and performance art. The Sitting Room, an intimate bistro-bar, is on its ground floor.

- Turn south on Roy one block to W. Mercer St. and Ozzie's Diner, a burger and pizza joint and karaoke bar. On its north wall a bizarre mural shows a quaint old-timey family, drinking peacefully out of doors. Three doors west of Ozzie's is the Streamline Tavern, a small, minimally cleaned up dive.

- Turn east on Mercer to Queen Anne Ave., the heart of the Lower Queen Anne business district (also known as Uptown). At the northeast corner of Queen Anne and Mercer, the MarQueen Hotel occupies a block-long brick former apartment building. Near the northwest corner, Peso's Mexican restaurant sports iconic wrought-iron art.

- Turn south on Queen Anne Ave. N. On this block are the Mecca Cafe (down-home cooking and strong drinks), the Uptown Espresso chain's flagship branch, the now-closed Uptown Theater, and the only Dick's Drive-In (Walks 15 and 25) to offer indoor seating. At Republican St., turn east and walk one block to 1st Ave. N., where two 1929 apartment buildings are now the Inn at Queen Anne.

- Go north on 1st. To your left are three popular restaurants, Floyd's Place (barbecue), Racha Noodles (Thai), and T. S. McHugh's (upmarket pub grub). At 1st and Mercer are a Metropolitan Market strip mall and Easy Street Records, heaven for indie-music lovers.

- Turn west on Roy. To your left is the modern arced A-frame of St. Paul's Episcopal Church. The parish has been around since 1892; this building was built in 1962 to coincide with the World's Fair. It sports a public garden with a circular concrete labyrinth.

- Continue on Roy to Queen Anne Ave. and Counterbalance Park, named in honor of the old cable-car line. In the 1980s, it was the site of a Dr. Seuss–esque restaurant building, which disapproving residents unofficially called "the blob."

- To return to your start, backtrack to the northeast corner of 1st and Mercer and take a #2 bus to 7th and Raye.

CONNECTING THE WALKS

This walk connects easily to two other walks. It ends near Walk 5. At Queen Anne Ave. and Republican you're four blocks north and three blocks northwest of Walk 7.

POINTS OF INTEREST

Seattle Church of Christ seattlechurchofchrist.org, 2555 8th Ave. W., 425-407-0582

Mt. Pleasant Cemetery 700 W. Raye St., 206-282-1270

Targy's 600 W. Crockett St., 206-352-8882

Queen Anne High School Condominiums 201 Galer St.

Kerry Park seattle.gov/parks, 211 W. Highland Dr.

On the Boards ontheboards.org, 100 W. Roy St., 206-217-9886

Ozzie's Diner ozziesseattle.com, 105 W. Mercer St., 206-284-4618

Peso's pesoskitchen.com, 605 Queen Anne Ave. N., 206-283-9353

Dick's Drive-In dicksdrivein.com, 500 Queen Anne Ave. N., 206-285-5155

St. Paul's Episcopal Church stpaulseattle. org, 15 Roy St., 206-282-0786

ROUTE SUMMARY

1. Start on 8th Ave. W., walking north from W. Halladay St.
2. Turn right on W. Raye St.
3. Turn south on 6th Ave. W.
4. Turn east on W. Crockett St.
5. Turn north on 4th Ave. W.
6. Turn east on W. McGraw St. Dogleg left and right on 1st Ave. N. back to McGraw.

Victoria Apartments

7. Continue east on McGraw five blocks to the street-end viewpoint east of Bigelow Ave. N.

8. Backtrack to Bigelow and turn south on Bigelow.

9. Turn west on Boston St.

10. Turn south on Queen Anne Ave. N. Continue to W. Galer St.

11. Take the steps east to 1st Ave. W. and Galer. Continue east on Galer.

12. Turn south on 2nd Ave. N., which bends west into Highland Drive.

13. Continue west on Highland.

14. Turn south on 7th Ave. W.

15. Dogleg onto Prospect St., then on to W. Kinnear Pl., then back to 7th.

16. Turn southeast on W. Olympic Pl., which bends east.

17. Turn south on 2nd Ave. W.

18. Turn east on W. Roy St.

19. Turn south on 1st Ave. W.

20. Turn east on W. Mercer St.

21. Turn south on Queen Anne Ave.

22. Turn east on Republican St.

23. Go north on 1st Ave. N.

24. Go west on Roy St. to Queen Anne Ave.

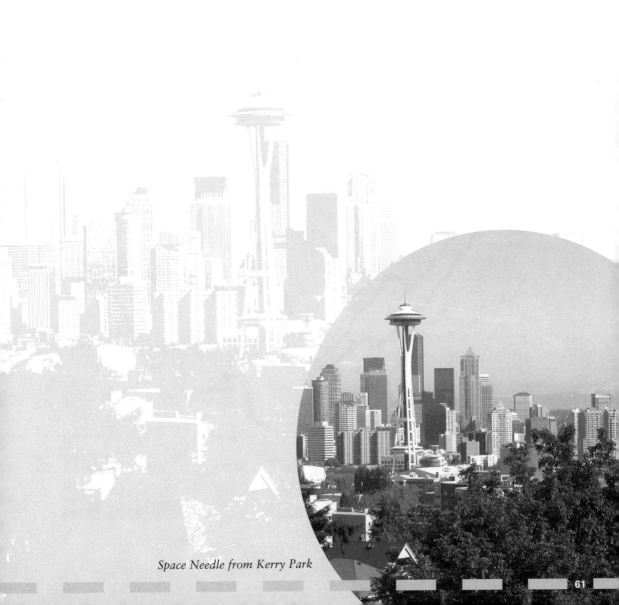

Space Needle from Kerry Park

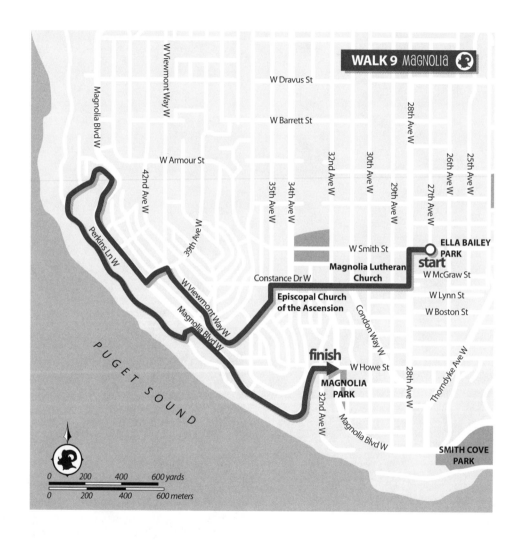

WALK 9 Magnolia

W Dravus St

W Barrett St

W Armour St

W Viewmont Way W

Magnolia Blvd W

42nd Ave W

39th Ave W

35th Ave W

34th Ave W

32nd Ave W

30th Ave W

29th Ave W

28th Ave W

27th Ave W

26th Ave W

25th Ave W

Perkins Ln W

W Viewmont Way W

Magnolia Blvd W

W Smith St

Magnolia Lutheran Church

ELLA BAILEY PARK

start

W McGraw St

Constance Dr W

Episcopal Church of the Ascension

Condon Way W

W Lynn St

W Boston St

finish

W Howe St

MAGNOLIA PARK

32nd Ave W

28th Ave W

Thorndyke Ave W

Magnolia Blvd W

SMITH COVE PARK

P U G E T S O U N D

0   200   400   600 yards
0   200   400   600 meters

9 Magnolia: MODERN MANSIONS AND MUDSLIDES

BOUNDARIES: 27th Ave. W., W. Smith St., Perkins Lane W., and Magnolia Blvd. W.
DISTANCE: 3¼ miles
DIFFICULTY: Moderate (one stairway)
PARKING: Free street parking
PUBLIC TRANSIT: Metro route #24 stops at 28th Ave. W. and W. McGraw St.

As the legend goes, while charting Puget Sound and its lands from his ship, British explorer George Vancouver spied some lovely magnolia trees rising atop a tall bluff on a peninsula at Elliott Bay's northern lip. Capt. Vancouver labeled that peninsula "Magnolia." The name stuck, even though explorations on land confirmed that those were really madrona trees. Yet the name "Magnolia," with its intimations of Southern gentility, fit what became a patrician village within the city, a home to spectacular views (and equally spectacular view homes, many sporting a more midcentury modern sense of style than those on neighboring Queen Anne Hill). Another Seattle neighborhood eventually got named "Madrona" (Walk 21).

● Start at Ella Bailey Park, 27th Ave. W. and W. Smith St. This recent addition to Seattle's park system reuses the playground of a now-closed school, and offers a great view of Elliott Bay and the downtown skyline.

● Turn west on Smith and continue for one block. Turn south on W. 28th St. Pass the handsome brick front of the shuttered Magnolia Elementary and the intersection with the eastbound W. McGraw St., and reach the intersection with the westbound (and noncontiguous) W. McGraw St.

● Walk west on McGraw, which at first is a solid middle-class residential street heading downhill toward 31st Ave. W. There you find Magnolia Lutheran's tall-pyramid spire, and a more unassuming Latter-Day Saints church across from it.

One block west at 32nd Ave. W., you've reached Magnolia Village, the neighborhood's shopping district. The sidewalks here are lined with real, albeit nonnative, magnolia trees. Book readers (a population I presume you are among) will enjoy the homey and inviting Magnolia's Bookstore. This is also your only opportunity along this walk to fill (or empty) your body. Among your choices here are Upper Crust Bakery, Village Pub, Swirl wine bar, Mexican cafe El Ranchon, and cozy Chinese restaurant and bar Gim Wah.

● Turn south on 35th Ave. W. for one block, toward the subdued Episcopal Church of the Ascension. Turn southwest on Viewmont Way W. As the streets here become curvier, the houses become fancier.

● At the intersection with Constance Dr. W., keep right. Viewmont Way W. here becomes West Viewmont Way W., winding northwest. (Seattle's street nomenclature, if you haven't already figured out, can have its quirks.) This street and those surrounding it are exceptionally wide, adding to the feeling of big-sky spaciousness.

● Turn southwest on W. Parkmont Pl. for two blocks; then turn northwest onto Magnolia Blvd. W. To your right, you pass big houses and small mansions in a wide variety of styles, from brick Tudor manors to suburban ranch houses on steroids. To your left, a long, grassy, public view corridor looks out toward the Olympic Peninsula and mountains, with benches and running paths and occasional make-out parking spots.

● At the fork with W. Raye St., turn left. Raye winds downhill through the Magnolia Bluff greenbelt. You've gone instantly from a controlled world of urban luxury into the illusion of being in a deep, wild forest, among tall trees and wild vines. (A word of caution: This stretch of Raye is a narrow two-lane road without sidewalks.)

● Raye ends at an intersection with Perkins Lane W. Turn southeast (left) on this curvy, one-lane road. Here the illusion of woodsy solitude is broken only by brief glimpses of the bay and by the driveways of residences, where urban hermits live in greater or lesser fear of mudslides. This fate occurred to several unlucky houses in the winter of 1996 to 1997. That part of Perkins has remained closed. Just before the concrete barriers marking the end of the road, climb a long set of concrete steps heading up the hillside back to Magnolia Blvd.

● Walk southeast on the west side of Magnolia Blvd., alongside the other walkers, runners, and bicyclists enjoying the street's park side. (The only people you're likely to see outside on the other side, the side with the big houses and the well-manicured shrubbery, are gardeners and couriers.) Peering over the bluff, you may see the remnants of a Perkins Lane mudslide-victim house. Magnolia Blvd. then bends north toward W. Howe St.

- Turn east on Howe, which becomes a short bridge over Pleasant Valley, a ravine between the peninsula's two hills. At the east end of this bridge is an intersection with a street that's labeled both Clise Pl. W. (northbound) and Magnolia Blvd. (southbound). The southwest corner of this intersection bears an entrance to Magnolia Park, a narrow, wooded park with an easy trail down to the bay.

- From here you have three options: Continue east on Howe four blocks to 28th (seven blocks south of this walk's start), continue on Howe three blocks to a #29 or 31 bus at 29th Ave. W., or take Clise north a quarter mile back to Magnolia Village.

CONNECTING THE WALKS

This walk connects easily to two other walks. At 35th Ave. W. and W. McGraw St., you're 1.3 miles south of Walk 10. From this walk's end, you can turn south on Magnolia Blvd. W., which bends east and leads to the Magnolia Bridge, down to Walk 7 (1.2 miles away).

POINTS OF INTEREST

Ella Bailey Park seatle.gov/parks, 27th Ave. W. and W. Smith St.

Magnolia Lutheran Church magnolialutheranchurch.com, 2414 31st Ave. W., 206-284-0155

Upper Crust Bakery uppercrustseattle.com, 3204 W. McGraw St., 206-283-1003

Magnolia's Bookstore 3206 W. McGraw St., 206-283-1062

Magnolia Village Pub magnolia-villagepub.com, 3221 W. McGraw St., 206-285-9756

Gim Wah 3418 W. McGraw St., 206-284-7000

Episcopal Church of the Ascension ascensionseattle.org, 2330 Viewmont Way W., 206-283-3967

Magnolia Park seatle.gov/parks, 1461 Magnolia Blvd. W.

route summary

1. Start at 27th Ave. W. and W. Smith St. Turn west on Smith.

2. Turn south on W. 28th St.

3. Turn west on W. McGraw St.

4. Turn south on 35th Ave. W.

5. Turn southwest on Viewmont Way W., which winds northwest.

6. Turn southwest on W. Parkmont Pl.

7. Turn northwest on Magnolia Blvd. W.

8. Turn left on W. Raye St., winding downhill.

9. Turn southeast on Perkins Lane W., to the steps leading back up to Magnolia Blvd.

10. Walk southeast on Magnolia Blvd., which bends north toward an intersection with W. Howe St.

11. Turn east on Howe two blocks, to the intersection with Clise Pl. W.

12. Either continue on Howe to 28th Ave. W., or take Clise Pl. north back to Magnolia Village.

Magnolia bluff

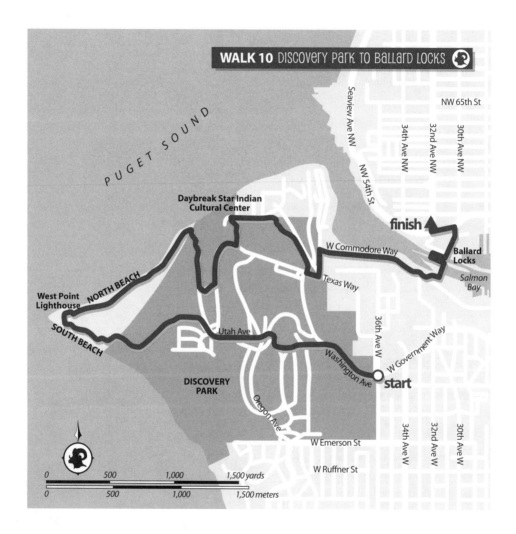

PUGET SOUND

Seaview Ave NW

NW 65th St

34th Ave NW

32nd Ave NW

30th Ave NW

NW 54th St

Daybreak Star Indian
Cultural Center

finish

W Commodore Way

Ballard
Locks

Texas Way

Salmon
Bay

West Point
Lighthouse

NORTH BEACH

SOUTH BEACH

Utah Ave

36th Ave W

W Government Way

Washington Ave

start

DISCOVERY
PARK

Oregon Ave

W Emerson St

34th Ave W

32nd Ave W

30th Ave W

W Ruffner St

| 0 | 500 | 1,000 | 1,500 yards |
| 0 | 500 | 1,000 | 1,500 meters |

10 Discovery Park to Ballard Locks: Army Issue

BOUNDARIES: 36th Ave. W., W. Government Way, Utah Ave., 32nd Ave. NW, and NW 54th St.
DISTANCE: 5 miles
DIFFICULTY: Difficult (one steep uphill trail)
PARKING: Free parking in Discovery Park east lot, just inside the Government Way entrance
PUBLIC TRANSIT: Metro route #33 stops at this walk's start.

Two of Seattle's most popular scenic spots are legacies from the US Army. The former Fort Lawton in northwest Magnolia, which Seattle gave the Army in 1900 and the Army returned to the city in 1972, is now Discovery Park. The city's biggest park encompasses 534 acres, mostly reclaimed for nature and nature-loving humans. It has walking trails ranging from flat to steep, and a restored lighthouse guarding a wide beachfront. Just north of Discovery, the Hiram M. Chittenden (a.k.a. Ballard) Locks, built in 1916 and managed by the Army Corps of Engineers, is the gateway between Lakes Union and Washington. A key passageway for both pleasure and commercial boats (and for our precious salmon), it also serves as a water-level footbridge across the Lake Washington Ship Canal, with finely landscaped grounds at both ends.

● Start at Discovery Park's east entrance, 36th Ave. W. and W. Government Way. Take the separate sidewalk to the south of the vehicular road.

● The first left turn you can take from here leads you, past a parking lot, to the Discovery Park Visitor Center. From there backtrack to, and continue westward on, Government Way, whose name changes to Washington Ave. in the old fort's naming system. This road is initially heavily wooded with mostly deciduous trees. At the top of a mild slope you reach a large clearing.

Continue as Washington Ave. bends northwest and then west again, past the Fort Lawton Historic District, two stretches of white-and-yellow painted wood buildings (including officers' residences, a chapel, a bus shelter, and a gym) separated by a huge open meadow (a great place for kite flying and running about). The Army still uses some of the buildings; these are fenced off. Amid these old wooden structures sits a piece of cold-war tech, a radar tower shaped like a giant golf ball.

- Washington Ave. bends south, then intersects with Oregon Ave. Turn north on Oregon toward an old, long bus shelter. (Like many of the old fort structures, it was a location in the 1973 James Caan movie *Cinderella Liberty*.) North of this shelter, turn left onto Utah Ave. It leads initially through a meadow with small trees and shrubs.

- Head west on this carless (except for official vehicles) road as it winds gently downhill, past the old fort stables, then past a 1950s suburban-style military housing tract (which may or may not be still standing as you read this). You might wish to hold your nose as you approach the West Point Treatment Plant. (At least they're scrubbing the city's wastewater now. They used to just pipe it out to sea.)

  Past the plant, the air turns to the aroma of saltwater as you approach the West Point Lighthouse, still warning ships after 130 years. The city undertook a major restoration of the brick-and-stucco building in 2009 to 2010. The point itself separates South Beach and North Beach.

- Turn east onto North Beach. Turn just inland from the beach onto a main dirt trail, which winds between the shore and the treatment plant's (mostly obscured by plants) north wall. This trail passes an

SIDE TRIP: SHILSHOLE AND GOLDEN GARDENS

For more Puget Sound scenery, keep walking west on the Burke-Gilman Trail beyond this walk's official end point at 32nd Ave. NW. The trail bends north along the shore. Within a half mile you're at the waterfront restaurant Ray's Boathouse, the start of the Shilshole strip. Another half mile and you're at the Shilshole Bay Marina, packed with docked pleasure boats and watched over by a statue of legendary explorer Leif Erikson. The trail ends another three-quarters of a mile north, at Golden Gardens Park. This long stretch of beach and forested hillside trails is popular year-round.

aquatic-bird habitat, a series of shallow ponds and marshes. At its end, the trail connects with a steep switchback path that bends uphill and back into the main park.

If you'd like an easier trod to and from the beach, follow this part of the walk in reverse, as follows: Where Utah Ave. bends northwest at the old subdivision homes, turn onto a side path that starts parallel at Utah's right side. This path bends north, to the steep path down the bluff to the beach. Turn southwest along the shoreline to the lighthouse. Turn east onto Utah, winding gently uphill back to the subdivision houses. Take a hard left back onto the northbound path you were just on. At your first chance, take two quick left turns. That will take you toward Daybreak Star, as noted below.

- At the top of the hill, the trail leading from the hill climb forks. Take the left (south-southeasterly) fork to another paved road. Beyond that, you find a concrete restroom structure to your left. Beyond that, turn left onto the Loop Trail. Take another left onto another paved road heading north.

This road takes you toward the southern side of the Daybreak Star Indian Cultural Center. The arts and educational facility was established in 1973 by the United Indians of All Tribes Foundation, after Native activists staged a 1970 sit-in on the soon-to-be-abandoned fort property. Take a left onto the center's grounds, around the striking angular building (resembling an eight-sided star) with tribal motifs within and without.

- Turn right on the road north of Daybreak Star, heading east then bending southeast. You're soon surrounded by another thickly forested area. See if you can spot some of the many small and large birds in the park (more than 200 different species, according to the Seattle Audubon Society). This unnamed road intersects with Texas Way. If you want to end your walk now, take a right onto Texas Way to a route #33 bus stop. Or you can turn south from that bus stop and onto Illinois Ave., which leads back to Washington Ave. and the park's east entrance.

- To continue with this walk's second leg, turn east (left) on Texas Way, then north on 40th Ave. W. and out of the park. Turn east onto W. Commodore Way. On its north side are some large waterfront homes, many equipped with their own private boat docks. Soon you pass under the lovely rust-colored iron lattice that is the BNSF

Railway's Salmon Bay Bridge. The 1914 drawbridge has a huge overhead counterweight on the north half of its single-truss superstructure.

- This bridge's southern approach lies at the western end of Commodore Park, part of the Ballard Locks' spiffy grounds. Take the paved walk past the bushes and flower beds, east to the locks.

- Within the lower level of the locks' pedestrian passage, a dark room with big picture windows looks in on the fish ladder, built into the locks to help salmon return to spawn. You can view the ladder from above when you walk up the short outdoor ramp to the roof. A sculpture here by Paul Sorey called *Salmon Waves* depicts metallic ocean waves swirling up.

- The fish ladder's roof is the entry to the locks' pedestrian passage. It takes you over the spillway structure, then, with swinging metal footbridges, across the two locks. Watch the boats enter the locks, whose water level is either filled or lowered. (The Corps of Engineers, which maintains the Lake Washington Ship Canal system, keeps the freshwater east of the locks 20 to 22 feet higher than the saltwater west of the locks.)

- On the north side of the locks, depending on which footbridges are open, you could be east or west of a concrete castle. It's the locks' office and visitor center, and it only happens to look like the Corps of Engineers' fortress logo. Take the sidewalk to its west, heading north through the Carl S. English Jr. Botanical Garden. The English-style garden holds more than 500 plant species from across the world.

- Take this paved walk north and out of the locks' grounds, to NW 54th St. To your right is the Lockspot, a quaint seafood grill and bar. One block to your left, at 32nd Ave. NW, is Totem House, a veteran fish-and-chips shop designed to imitate a Northwest tribal longhouse. The local Red Mill hamburger chain recently took over the space, serving Totem House's seafood specialties, as well as Red Mill's burgers.

- One block north of there, at 32nd and NW Market Street, is a stop for bus route #17 to downtown.

CONNECTING THE WALKS

This walk connects easily to two other walks. It starts 1.3 miles north of Walk 9 and ends a half mile west of Walk 13.

POINTS OF INTEREST

Discovery Park Visitor Center seattle.gov/parks, 3801 W. Government Way, 206-386-4236

West Point Lighthouse foot of Utah Ave. in Discovery Park, 206-386-4236

Daybreak Star Indian Cultural Center unitedindians.org, northwest end of Discovery Park, 206-285-4425

Ballard (Hiram M. Chittenden) Locks nws.usace.army.mil, 3015 NW 54th St., 206-783-7059

Lockspot Cafe 3005 NW 54th St., 206-789-4865

Red Mill Burgers at the Totem House redmillburgers.com, 3058 NW 54th St.

ROUTE SUMMARY

1. Start at W. Government Way walking west from 36th Ave. W. into Discovery Park, where it becomes Washington Ave.

2. Washington Ave. bends south, then intersects with Oregon Ave. Turn west to Utah Ave. and take a left.

3. Follow Utah Ave. downhill to the West Point Lighthouse.

4. Turn east along North Beach, then follow the main trail. This trail bends uphill and back into the main park.

5. At the top of the hill, take the left trail heading south-southeast.

6. Just beyond a restroom building, take a left onto the Loop Trail.

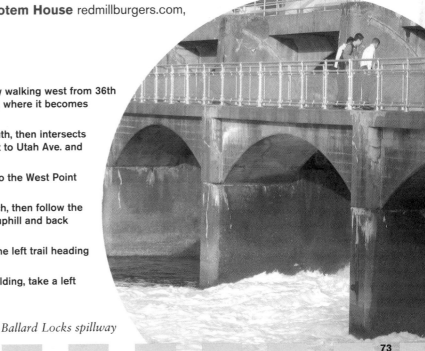

Ballard Locks spillway

7. Take another left onto a paved road heading north, toward the Daybreak Star Indian Cultural Center.

8. Take a left onto the center's grounds to its north side.

9. Turn east on the main road north of Daybreak Star, which bends southeast, finally intersecting with Texas Way.

10. To end your walk here, turn west on Texas Way to a bus stop, then either take a #33 bus or walk south on Illinois Ave. back to Washington Ave.

11. To continue with this walk, turn east on Texas Way.

12. Turn north on 40th Ave. W. out of the park.

13. Turn east on W. Commodore Way to the Ballard (Hiram M. Chittenden) Locks.

14. Cross the locks' pedestrian passageway across the Lake Washington Ship Canal.

15. Take the paved path north and out of the locks' grounds.

16. Turn left on NW 54th St. to 32nd Ave. NW.

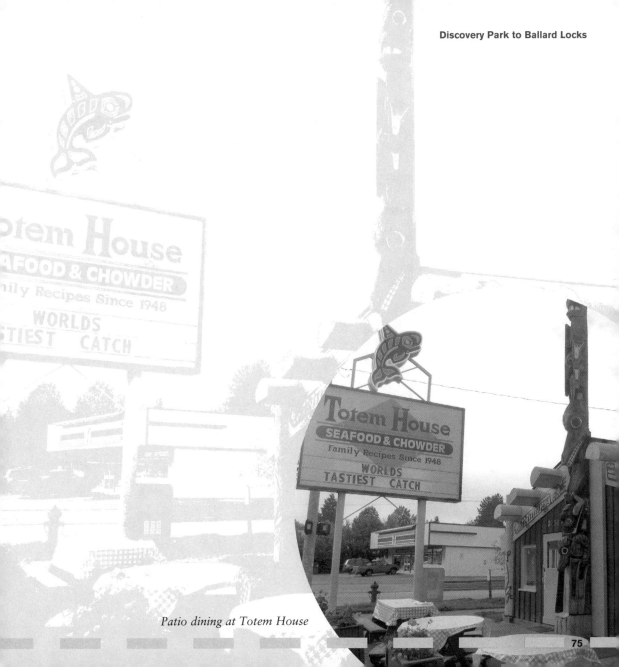

Patio dining at Totem House

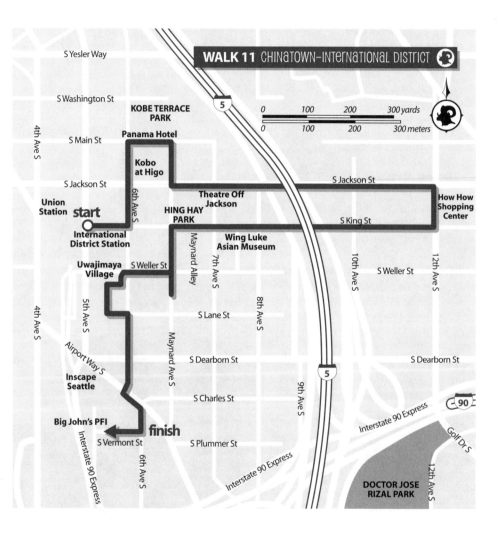

S Yesler Way

S Washington St

S Main St

S Jackson St

4th Ave S

KOBE TERRACE PARK

Panama Hotel

Kobo at Higo

6th Ave S

I-5

0   100   200   300 yards
0   100   200   300 meters

S Jackson St

Theatre Off Jackson

HING HAY PARK

S King St

How How Shopping Center

Union Station

start

International District Station

Uwajimaya Village

S Weller St

Maynard Alley

7th Ave S

Wing Luke Asian Museum

10th Ave S

S Weller St

12th Ave S

5th Ave S

Maynard Ave S

S Lane St

8th Ave S

4th Ave S

Airport Way S

Inscape Seattle

S Dearborn St

9th Ave S

S Dearborn St

I-5

Big John's PFI

finish

S Vermont St

6th Ave S

S Charles St

S Plummer St

Interstate 90 Express

I-90

Interstate 90 Express

Interstate 90 Express

Golf Dr S

DOCTOR JOSE RIZAL PARK

12th Ave S

11 CHINATOWN-INTERNATIONAL DISTRICT: "PAN-ASIAN" BEFORE THAT WAS A WORD

BOUNDARIES: **5th Ave. S., 12th Ave. S., S. Main St., and S. Vermont St.**
DISTANCE: **1¾ miles**
DIFFICULTY: **Easy (one brief incline)**
PARKING: **Limited metered street parking; pay lots and garages include the Uwajimaya Village lot, 600 5th Ave. S.**
PUBLIC TRANSIT: **Seattle Transit Tunnel International District Station; a dozen Metro routes stop at 5th Ave. S. and S. Jackson St.**

This region would not have become what it is without the vital contributions of Chinese American railway workers, Japanese American farmers, and Filipino American cannery workers—contributions that have *not* always been appreciated. White militants in 1886 staged anti-Chinese riots, rounding up 350 people and ordering them at gunpoint to board the next steamship out of town. During World War II, Japanese Americans throughout the Pacific states were sent to internment camps. Through it all, the neighborhood east of Pioneer Square has remained the spiritual home of Asian Seattle. In recent decades, Vietnamese immigrants have added their own dimensions to this exciting mélange of languages, architectures, and decorative styles.

● Start outside the Transit Tunnel's International District Station at 5th Ave. S. and S. King St. To your west is neoclassical Union Station, the larger of Seattle's two heritage railway stations. Its restored lobby is a rental party space.

● South of Union Station, Paul Allen has built four neo-modern midrise buildings. If you didn't know about Allen's sci-fi appreciation (he named his company "Vulcan"), you can tell by the big air vents at 5th and Weller, between two of Allen's buildings. They look like abstracted versions of *Doctor Who*'s archvillains, the Daleks.

● Cross 5th. As you reach King St., walk under an elaborate 45-foot Chinese archway built in 2008. Walk east along King one block to 6th Ave. S. At the northeast corner, a hostel occupies the 1925 American Hotel. At the southeast corner, the Pink Gorilla store offers vintage video games.

- Turn north on 6th and continue for two blocks. At 6th and S. Jackson St., a branch of Washington Federal Savings sports a mansard roof with Chinese-inspired red tile; its front sports a mural portrait of eight Chinese "immortals."

Across Jackson, the Higo five-and-ten store is now Kobo, a crafts gallery and home-furnishings store. North of Jackson, the 1903 Main Street School Annex was Seattle's first kindergarten; the small wood-frame building is now offices. It's across from the 1914 NP Hotel, now low-income apartments.

- Turn east onto S. Main St., at a neon rice bowl outside a now-closed cafe. This segment goes steeply uphill, but only for one block. Halfway up the block, the 1910 Panama Hotel contains a teahouse and a private museum (open by appointment) remembering the Japanese American community before the World War II internment. Across the street, Kobe Terrace Park includes a community garden rising up a hillside, with a 200-year-old stone lantern at its top.

- Turn south on Maynard Ave. S. back to Jackson. The Far East Building shows the result of a 1908 street regrade; what are now its street-level storefronts were built beneath what had been two separate buildings. At the southwest corner, the 1915 Bush Hotel now has four floors of low-income apartments above two floors of retail and community-organization offices.

- Turn east on Jackson. Just east of 6th, the Asia Bar-B-Que entices with roasted chickens hanging in the window. At Maynard Ave. S., *Heaven, Man, and Earth* is a 12-foot abstract bronze sculpture by local artist George Tsutakawa. Just south of the southwest corner of Jackson and Maynard Ave. S., Theatre Off Jackson stages plays and screens films in a 1915-era garage.

Continue along the north side of Jackson under the I-5 freeway overpass pillars, painted red and gold with Native American fish icons. Just beyond the freeway is the Pacific Rim Center, a condo-retail box anchored by the New Hong Kong Restaurant.

Continue toward 12th Ave. S., now the main drag of Seattle's Vietnamese community. It used to be the center of a thriving jazz scene, centered in bars and private after-hours clubs. This history is noted in a small free-standing plaque near 12th and Jackson's northwest corner.

● Turn south on 12th, past the four-story How How Shopping Center.

● Turn west on King, through a largely industrial block. On King's north side, Acme Farms is one of the state's leading poultry processing firms. (Its equipment kills birds more successfully than that of a certain fictional Acme.) At 10th Ave. S., the King Street Southern Baptist Church and Chinese Southern Baptist Mission is a small, solid red brick box with Gothic stained-glass windows.

● Continue along King under the freeway pillars, with King Street Station's clock tower (Walk 1) in front of you. At 8th and King, the 1910 East Kong Yick Building houses the Wing Luke Asian Museum, which calls itself the only "pan-Asian Pacific American museum" in the United States. Across King, the Bing Kung Association (a "tong" or fraternal organization aiding immigrants) features a tiled balcony on its fourth floor, with a Masonic logo in relief above it. (The building once housed a Masonic temple.)

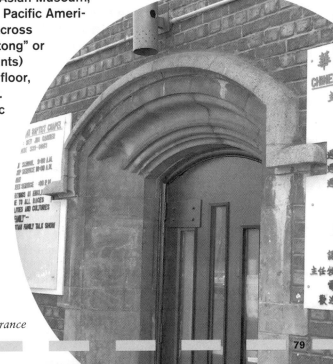

On the south side of King between 7th Ave. S. and Maynard is Maynard Alley. You can see the green-painted wall and boarded-up entrance to Wah Mee, a private gambling club dating to the 1920s. In 1983 it was the site of Washington State's worst mass murder when three robbers shot 14 people, killing all but one.

Chinese Southern Baptist Church entrance

At King and Maynard, the 1909 Rex Hotel houses Tai Tung, the neighborhood's oldest continually operating restaurant (since 1935). It's kitty-corner from Hing Hay Park, with an elaborate multicultural mural and a grand Chinese pavilion (made in Taiwan).

● Turn south on Maynard. Just south of King, a round window with red and black brick "sunbeams" marks the Eastern Hotel. It was built in 1911 by a company founded in 1868 by Chin Chun Hock, probably Seattle's first Chinese settler. It now has a mini-museum honoring Filipino writer Carlos Bulosan, who once lived here. It also houses the Seattle Pinball Museum, a storefront filled with restored American flipper games. For a $7.50 admission fee, you can play for as long as you can stand the noise.

Just south of the Eastern is the Sing Keong Society (another Chinese "benevolent association"), with a pagoda-style false front. South of S. Weller St., observe the Bush Garden Japanese restaurant's simple stone-and-bamboo facade. It's more exquisite on the inside.

● Backtrack a half block to Maynard and Weller. Turn west on Weller and walk one block, past the Ocean City Restaurant's elaborate storefront. At 6th and Weller, Ming's Art Gallery occupies part of the blue-tile-roofed ex-home of the Uwajimaya Japanese market. Uwajimaya Village, the store's current complex, is across Weller to your left.

● Enter and view the shops at Uwajimaya Village's north side, starting with the Kinokuniya Book Store. It has many beautiful gift items even if you don't read the language. Head out the bookstore's south doors into a mall area, then into the Uwajimaya store itself. It offers food, fashions, home decor, cookware, toys, and gifts. Exit through the store's south entrance; turn east back to 6th Ave. S. at S. Lane St.

● Turn south on 6th. On the east side, a new low-rise commercial building includes Daiso, the Japanese equivalent of a dollar store (most items here range from $1.50 to $2). You reach the end of 6th at a diagonal intersection with Airport Way S., in front of the former US Immigrant Station and Assay Office. Thousands of new citizens came through this neoclassical edifice from 1932 to 2004. Some stayed for weeks or months, jailed under the Chinese Exclusion Act (effective from 1882 through 1943) before they could join relatives already living in the United States. The 77,000-square-foot building reopened in 2010 as Inscape, a complex of artist studios and exhibit spaces. One of its tenants is the Northwest Museum of Legends and Lore, with exhibits related to paranormal activity, UFOs, Bigfoot, ghosts, and related topics.

● Cross Airport and turn southeast. The boxy modern building next to the ex-immigration complex is the former site of the Lawrimore Project, an art installation space. Take a dogleg right turn back onto 6th for one block, to the large brick warehouse at S. Vermont St. At that building's left end is Big John's PFI (a.k.a. Pacific Food Importers), a bulk-foods outlet with European cheeses, meats, olive oils, and pasta.

● Backtrack to Airport, walk northwest to 5th, and turn north back to your start.

CONNECTING THE WALKS

This walk connects easily to four other walks. It starts one block south and three blocks east of Walk 1, and eight blocks from Walk 2. It ends one block north and five blocks east of Walk 12. At 12th and Jackson you're six blocks west of Walk 28.

POINTS OF INTEREST

Kobo at Higo koboseattle.com, 604 S. Jackson St., 206-381-3000

Panama Hotel Tea & Coffee House panamahotel.net, 607 S. Main St., 206-515-4000

Kobe Terrace Park seattle.gov/parks, 221 6th Ave. S.

Theatre Off Jackson theatreoffjackson.org, 409 7th Ave. S., 206-340-1049

Wing Luke Asian Museum wingluke.org, 707 S. King St., 206-623-5124

Tai Tung 659 S. King St., 206-622-7372

Bush Garden bushgarden.net, 614 Maynard Ave. S., 206-682-6830

Uwajimaya uwajimaya.com, 600 5th Ave. S., 206-624-6248

Inscape inscapearts.org, 815 Airport Way S., 206-257-3022

Big John's PFI bigjohnspfiseattle.com, 1001 6th Ave. S., 206-682-2022

route summary

1. Start on S. King St., walking east from 5th Ave. S.
2. Turn north on 6th Ave. S.
3. Turn east on S. Main St.
4. Turn south on Maynard Ave. S.
5. Turn east on S. Jackson St.
6. Turn south on 12th Ave. S.
7. Turn west on S. King St.
8. Turn south on Maynard Ave. S., to a half block south of S. Weller St.
9. Backtrack to Maynard and Weller.
10. Turn west on Weller back to 6th.
11. Turn south on 6th.
12. Turn southeast on Airport Way S.
13. Dogleg south back onto 6th and turn south to S. Vermont St.
14. Backtrack to Airport Way and walk northwest.
15. Turn north at 5th Ave. S., back to your start.

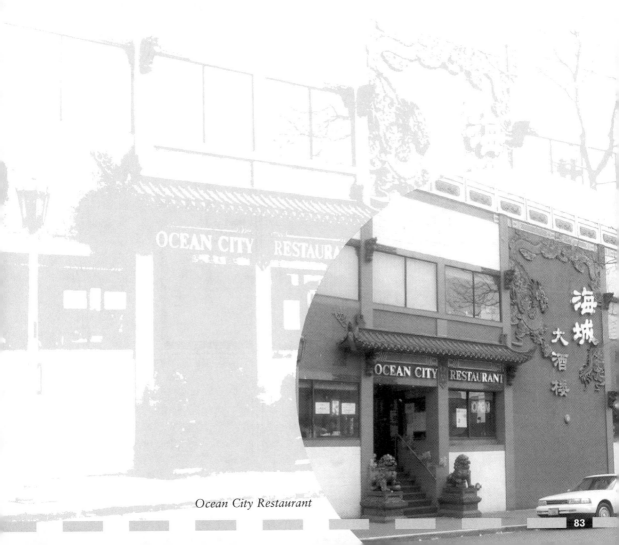

Ocean City Restaurant

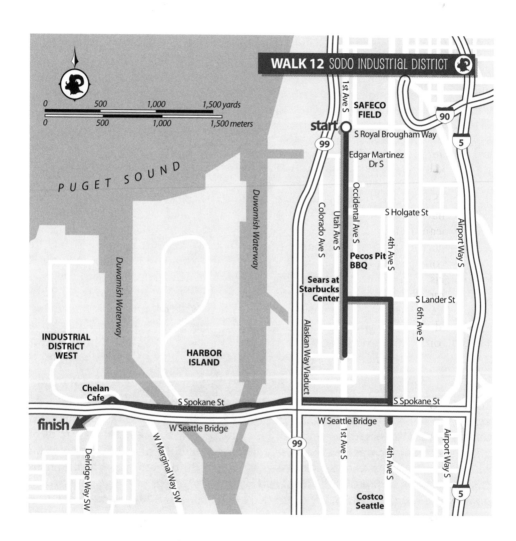

1st Ave S

SAFECO FIELD

start

S Royal Brougham Way

99

90

5

Edgar Martinez Dr S

Occidental Ave S

S Holgate St

Utah Ave S

Colorado Ave S

4th Ave S

Airport Way S

Pecos Pit BBQ

Sears at Starbucks Center

S Lander St

S 6th Ave S

Alaskan Way Viaduct

PUGET SOUND

Duwamish Waterway

Duwamish Waterway

INDUSTRIAL DISTRICT WEST

HARBOR ISLAND

Chelan Cafe

S Spokane St

S Spokane St

finish

W Seattle Bridge

W Seattle Bridge

99

1st Ave S

4th Ave S

Airport Way S

5

Delridge Way SW

W Marginal Way SW

Costco Seattle

0   500   1,000   1,500 yards
0   500   1,000   1,500 meters

12 SODO INDUSTRIAL DISTRICT: THEY STILL MAKE THINGS HERE

BOUNDARIES: S. Royal Brougham Way, 4th Ave. S., Chelan Ave. SW, and SW Spokane St.
DISTANCE: 4 miles, in two segments
DIFFICULTY: Easy (almost entirely flat)
PARKING: Pay lots and garages include the official Safeco Field and Qwest Field garages, which are emptier on non-game days.
PUBLIC TRANSIT: Link Light Rail Stadium Station; Metro routes #21, 22, 56, and 57

"TIDE LANDS HAS RIZ!" Early Seattle real-estate speculator H. H. Richardson chanted and printed that slogan to promote land sales in the then-underwater lands south of Pioneer Square. He meant these properties were rising in value, because they would eventually rise above sea level. Richardson's prophecies proved correct when dirt from the Denny Regrade (Walk 5) and other projects turned these wetlands high, dry, and ready for industry. Later promoters christened the area "SoDo," for "south of the Kingdome." After there was no more Kingdome, the acronym's meaning was changed to "south of downtown." This bastion of working-class values has been mostly protected from redevelopment by city zoning regulations, intended to preserve industrial businesses and their living-wage jobs. Along these wide, flat avenues you'll see a variety of structures made for the making and storing of a variety of things. The structures range from the new and functional to the weathered and gorgeous.

● **Start at the northwest entrance to Safeco Field, on the east side of 1st Ave. S. south of S. Royal Brougham Way. The older of the Kingdome's two replacement stadia, it's been home to the Mariners baseball team since 1999. Even when the team's not so hot, the stadium (with its high-tech retractable roof) is one of baseball's snazziest. Across 1st, the Pyramid Alehouse is the showcase pub for one of the region's biggest specialty brewers. (Royal Brougham Way was originally Connecticut St. In the 1980s it was rechristened in honor of a *Post-Intelligencer* sportswriter who died with his figurative boots on, in the Kingdome press box during a Seahawks football game.)**

- Walk south, past Safeco Field's even grander southwest entrance at 1st and Edgar Martinez Dr. S. (a single block of S. Atlantic St., renamed for the Mariners' former designated hitter). On the following block, a tall, narrow, handsome old brick industrial building stands watch over a block that's largely been razed for surface parking lots.

- South of S. Massachusetts St. are the Showbox SoDo music club and a wine shop in a former Murphy Bed factory. South of the latter is the Hooverville bar, named for the Depression-era shantytown that was near here. Beyond S. Holgate St., a huge and usually empty Krispy Kreme snack shop stands as an icon of yesterday's next big thing. South of that stands the gallery of wildlife and nature photographer Art Wolfe.

- South of S. Walker St., a white warehouse building houses Outdoor Research, a store selling serious camping and hiking clothes and gear. At S. Stacy St., a onetime gas station is the Pecos Pit BBQ stand, a sandwich shop with no indoor seating (just a couple of picnic tables outside) and sometimes-huge lines for its tender meats smothered in sauce. Down the next block is a popular Vietnamese cafe, Pho Cyclo.

Looking west, spy the green eyes of a cartoon mermaid peering from a 1907 brick clock tower. Cross to the west side of 1st for a closer look at Starbucks Center, the coffee giant's world headquarters. Seattle's largest commercial building by square footage, it was originally a Sears catalog warehouse. In 1925, the then catalog-only company built its second-ever retail store on the building's south side. It's now Sears' oldest existing store, buffeted by Office Max and Home Depot.

Adjacent to Home Depot at S. Lander St. is a finely aged low-rise featuring a Greek restaurant and a military surplus and hiking-gear store. Past S. Forest St. is Island Life, a hip tiki and bamboo furnishings store.

- At S. Hanford St., you've got lovingly restored midcentury kitsch at the K. R. Trigger and Vertigo buildings. Dentist and developer Scott Andrews bought these warehouses in the 1990s. He attracted architectural firms and other aesthetically minded tenants with such amenities as a gallery of classic neon signs. Cross 1st at the south side of Hanford, toward two more Andrews-developed wooden buildings. One of these, Sodo Park, is a rental reception space.

- Backtrack north along the east side of 1st. Just across Forest is an example of Seattle-First National Bank's handsome old branch design, still occupied by Bank of America. At the southeast corner of 1st and Lander, peer in at vintage signs at Western Neon. At the northeast corner with Lander, a classic wooden barn–style warehouse has housed a series of home-furnishings stores for more than six decades; its current tenant is Pius Kitchen & Bath.

- Turn east on Lander, toward 4th Ave. S. On 4th's north side, Jones Barbecue offers all the specialties of an authentic BBQ joint plus inside seats. On the south side, Pacific Galleries operates a huge antique mall and auction house.

- Turn south on the east side of 4th. The first building you encounter is the art deco yet utilitarian quarters of Esquin Wine Merchants. At 4th and Forest, across from Seattle's last Denny's franchise, the always-joyful pink neon of an Elephant Car Wash (Walk 5) stands adjacent to the Rabanco Recycling plant's loading platform. There, you can see huge piles of printed matter go to the great beyond.

  Orient Express, at 4th and Hanford, is a Chinese restaurant and lounge in a collection of old rail passenger cars previously known for decades as Andy's Diner. The Spanish suburban–style Fire Station #14, with two firefighter-training towers in back, has stood guard at 4th and Hanford since 1927. Western Bridge, a major contemporary art space, is hidden in a plain white building behind Gull Oil's offices south of S. Hinds St., but is definitely worth looking for. (Hint: It's across from the Siren Tavern's neon bull's-eye.)

- A bigger neon attraction awaits on the west side of 4th south of S. Spokane St., the giant white and pink CITY LIGHT letters on an electric substation. You could end your walk here, taking a Metro bus at the northeast corner of 4th and Spokane back to Safeco Field. Or, you could continue south on 4th for another half mile, past the substation's lovely lattice towers, to Costco Wholesale's original megastore.

- If you're continuing with this walk, backtrack to 4th and Spokane. Turn west onto the north side of Spokane. Be warned: This sidewalk, in the shadow of an auto-only viaduct and lined by rental-truck lots and loading docks, is lonely.

That all changes once you're west of East Marginal Way S. Here, you get a wide pedestrian and bicycle path separated from the roadway and lined with grass border strips and occasional trees. As it crosses the Duwamish Waterway's east fork, it offers a sequence of three sheltered viewpoints looking out to the harbor. (You can fish here; just don't eat your catch.) This path leads onto Harbor Island, built for industry in 1909 from fill dirt poured into the Duwamish delta. It's now mostly container docks, but you can still see the former Dutch Boy paint plant (now run by a Japanese firm) and the mammoth grain elevators of the defunct Fisher Flouring Mill.

● While you're on Harbor Island, cross SW Spokane St. at the first available crosswalk at the intersection with SW Manning St. Enter the pedestrian and bicycle lane on Spokane's south side. This will get you across the (lower) West Seattle Bridge, across the Duwamish's west fork.

● Once you're back on land, follow the ALKI TRAIL signs on the path as it turns northwest from Spokane to SW Marginal Pl., then cross three short crosswalks onto Chelan Ave. SW, north of Spokane. Your reward for a well-trod walk is a bite and/or sip at the Chelan Cafe, a venerable working folks' lunch spot. Just west of there, another trio of crosswalks gets you to a bus stop. Take route #21, 22, or 56 back to your start.

CONNECTING THE WALKS

This walk connects easily to three other walks. It starts one long block south of Walk 1, and it ends at the same place as Walk 34. Following the Alki Trail past this walk's end will get you (after 1¾ miles) to Walk 33.

POINTS OF INTEREST

Safeco Field mariners.mlb.com, 1250 1st Ave. S., 206-346-4001

Pecos Pit BBQ 2260 1st Ave. S., 206-623-0629

Sears at Starbucks Center sears.com, 76 S. Lander St., 206-344-4835

Island Life island-life.com, 2909 1st Ave. S., 206-340-1212

Pacific Galleries pacgal.com, 241 S. Lander St., 206-292-3999

Orient Express 2963 4th Ave. S., 206-682-0683

Costco costco.com, 4401 4th Ave. S., 206-674-1220

Chelan Cafe 3527 Chelan Ave. SW, 206-932-7383

route summary

1. Start at 1st Ave. S., walking south from S. Royal Brougham Way.
2. At S. Hanford St., turn around and backtrack north on 1st.
3. Turn east on S. Lander St.
4. Turn south on 4th Ave S.
5. Turn west on S. Spokane St.
6. Take the pedestrian and bicycle lane at the north side of the Spokane Street Bridge westbound, onto Harbor Island.
7. Cross Spokane at SW Manning St.
8. Take the pedestrian and bicycle lane at the south side of the (lower) West Seattle Bridge.
9. Turn right from Spokane onto W. Marginal Way SW, then onto Chelan Ave. SW.

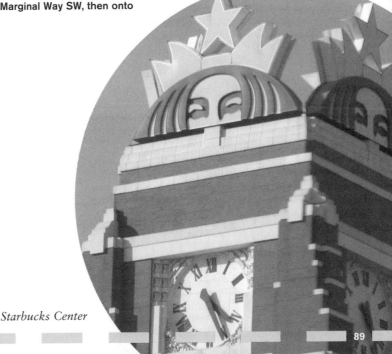

Starbucks Center

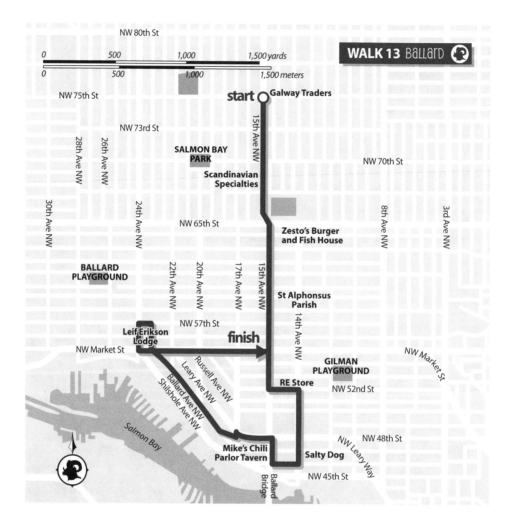

NW 80th St

0   500   1,000   1,500 yards

0   500   1,000   1,500 meters

NW 75th St

start

Galway Traders

NW 73rd St

28th Ave NW

26th Ave NW

15th Ave NW

SALMON BAY PARK

Scandinavian Specialties

NW 70th St

8th Ave NW

3rd Ave NW

30th Ave NW

24th Ave NW

NW 65th St

Zesto's Burger and Fish House

BALLARD PLAYGROUND

22nd Ave NW

20th Ave NW

17th Ave NW

15th Ave NW

St Alphonsus Parish

14th Ave NW

NW 57th St

Leif Erikson Lodge

finish

NW Market St

Russell Ave NW

Leary Ave NW

Ballard Ave NW

Shilshole Ave NW

GILMAN PLAYGROUND

NW Market St

RE Store

NW 52nd St

Salmon Bay

NW 48th St

NW Leary Way

Mike's Chili Parlor Tavern

Salty Dog

Ballard Bridge

NW 45th St

13 Ballard: Ya Sure, Ya Betcha!

BOUNDARIES: NW 75th St., 24th Ave. NW, Ballard Ave. NW, NW 46th St., and 14th Ave. NW
DISTANCE: 3½ miles
DIFFICULTY: Easy (flat or downhill)
PARKING: Free street parking
PUBLIC TRANSIT: Metro route #15 stops at this walk's start.

A local bumper sticker in the mid-2000s read, "We in Ballard welcome our new condo overlords." The sticker was sold by Archie McPhee, a novelty store that later moved to Wallingford (Walk 15). Archie's left a neighborhood that had originally developed around fishing, sawmills, and Scandinavian immigrant families. Having mostly survived the condo onslaught, it's now a quiet bedroom community, the spiritual home of the Seattle and Alaska fishing fleet, a quaint arts and shopping spot, and a happening nightlife zone. We start with the residential section (with some ethnic shopping and a couple twists on all-American dining), then join a historic cobblestoned main street before ending up in the neighborhood's more modern main drag.

- Start on the east side of 15th Ave. NW, north of NW 75th St., at Galway Traders, selling "pan-Celtic" food, clothing, books, and gifts. It's in a 1912 bungalow; the house's Irish-American builder carved shamrocks into the eaves.

- Walk south on 15th. This street has some fairly unique eateries. The first is Rizzo's French Dip cafe. (That's the only item on the menu.) Scandinavian Specialties, an unassuming storefront north of NW 67th St., is packed with Norse gifts and foods (packaged, take-out, or eat-in). The block after that belongs to Ballard High School, home to the fighting Ballard Beavers.

  At 15th and NW 65th St., Zesto's Burger and Fish House is a neighborhood institution, the former franchise of a now-defunct chain. At NW 58th St., St. Alphonsus Parish's sleek, modern curves provide a fine contrast to the parish school behind it, an Edwardian brick schoolhouse.

- Turn left on NW 52nd St. in front of Louie's Cuisine of China. Look to the north side of 52nd for a mural of a dark-skinned earth goddess staring back at you. It draws you toward the RE Store, vendors of used building materials, furnishings, and decor. East of that stands a bold neon sign exhorting you to ADD BARDAHL. It marks the headquarters of Bardahl Oil, makers of motor-oil additives and related products since the 1930s. The building's clad in green plastic paneling, a midcentury style that hasn't come back into fashion.

- Turn south on 14th Ave. NW. At 14th and NW Leary Way, you can easily miss Mars Hill Church, a black warehouse building with minimal signage. Inside is a contemporary megachurch that markets the Evangelical faith to the young and hip. At NW 46th St. you have an easier time finding the Salty Dog art and pottery studio; its front sports a mural of a theater curtain.

- Turn west on 46th to the Ballard Blocks retail project. Devised at the peak of the real-estate boom, it's two hulking big-box structures. Walk west past its central corridor to view "the Ballard spite house," a small bungalow whose elderly owner refused to sell to the developers. (She died before the completion of Ballard Blocks, which was built around her property.)

- Turn north on 15th to Mike's Chili Parlor Tavern. This working folks' pub with working folks' grub has been owned by the same family for nearly nine decades. Its brick-and-neon storefront proves deco-derived design can be manly. Continue on 15th one more block, then turn west on NW Leary Way, under the Ballard Bridge's northern end. The 1917-built double drawbridge over the Lake Washington Ship Canal is a great half-mile walk by itself. At its southern end is Fisherman's Terminal, home to the Seattle and Alaska fishing fleet.

- If you're continuing with this walk, keep going west on Leary. Look on Leary's south side for another vintage neon sign, promoting Craig's Auto Springs. Near 17th Ave. NW, a neon horse head sticks out from the 1940s wooden shed housing the 2 Bit Saloon.

- Take a dogleg south on 17th to NW 48th St.; then turn west on 48th to Ballard Ave. NW and hang a right, turning northwest into the Ballard Ave. historic district. For decades, these six blocks of old bars, hardware stores, and residential hotels were mostly preserved by neglect. In recent years, it's become a site for nightlife and art.

For your first block, you see some surviving machine shops and paint warehouses. Just beyond NW Dock St., Bad Albert's Tap & Grill marks the start of the bar-and-shopping strip. Across from it is OKOK, a gallery and "designer toy" boutique.

At the northeast corner of Ballard and NW Ione Pl., local celebrity chef Kathy Casey has her deli and wine shop. Next to that is the Conor Byrne Pub and its antique wooden back bar. Next to that is the Lock and Keel, a nautical-themed bar and BBQ joint with a 30-foot rowboat hanging from the ceiling. Next to that, Monster Art and Clothing stands behind an ornate 1893 facade.

Beyond 20th Ave. NW, King's Hardware starts a string of bars. They're anchored by the Tractor Tavern, a venerable live-music club. Northwest from there, drinkers at Hattie's Hat and the Old Town Alehouse are often found peeping across the street at a 1910 Elks building, where Olympic Health Club members toil behind big picture windows day and night.

Ballard Ave. then becomes a casual diner's dream, offering French cuisine, deluxe sandwiches, and sushi. There's funky shopping, too, including shoes, modern and retro furniture, fashion jewelry, garden accessories, hand-made European toys, and musical instruments.

The northeast corner of Ballard and 22nd Ave. NW is a pocket park called Marvin's Garden. It's a concrete patio with benches, anchored

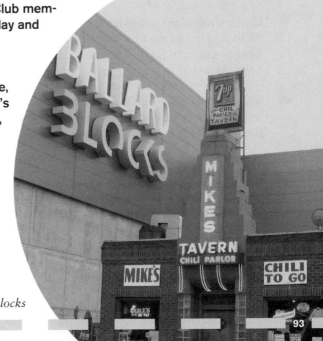

Mike's Chili Parlor Tavern and Ballard Blocks

by a short, new bell tower enclosing the half-ton brass bell from the old Ballard City Hall. It was named for Marvin Sjoberg, a colorful local character and self-proclaimed "mayor of Ballard" (decades after Seattle annexed the former independent town). The block continues with live music at the Sunset Tavern, drinks and German grub at the People's Pub, ethnic eats at Thai Ku and La Carta de Oaxaca, and swank food and drink at BelMar. Ballard Ave. bends north just before it ends at NW Market St.

- Turn west on Market, passing the snazzy Snoose Junction Pizzeria, to 24th Ave. NW. Head north on the east side of 24th, past the used fashion and furniture store Classic Consignment and a particularly massive big-box condo.

- Turn right onto the south side of NW 57th St., around the side of that big-box condo. Just east of it stands Leif Erikson Lodge. The chalet-inspired structure looks like a modernized old building; it only dates to 1984, the third building to house local Sons of Norway and Daughters of Norway. (The first, now Raisbeck Performance Hall, is on Walk 6.) At the lodge's east side, turn south and cut through a bank parking lot to NW 56th St.

- Cross a midblock crosswalk at 56th; take a marked sidewalk through another parking lot to Ballard Square (a former J. C. Penney divvied into smaller spaces). Descend the interior stairs to Ballard Square's main floor, and exit the building's south side back onto Market.

- Walk east on Market. On the north side of Market at 22nd is the Ballard Building, built in 1927 to house an Eagles lodge and a silent movie theater; the stately white structure now hosts offices and a gym.

On the south side of Market at 22nd is Bergen Place park, dedicated to the neighborhood's Nordic heritage. Next to it is Vera's Restaurant, a classic breakfast and lunch diner. On the north side of Market east of 22nd are Cupcake Royale, local ground zero of the gourmet-cupcake boom, and the Majestic Bay Theater, a triplex cinema "restored" in 2000 from a 1915 neighborhood movie house. (If any of the original building remains, I can't see it.) Beyond that is a stoic 1905 library building, which most recently housed a French restaurant.

East of 20th Ave. NW on the north side of Market lies the Ballard Blossom Shop with its elegant black, white, and neon facade. East of that is the Old Pequliar, an Irish pub that used to be a Swedish pub called the Valhalla. Across from there is Egan's, an intimate jazz and supper club.

● At the northwest corner of 15th and Market, pay your respects to the demolished Sunset Bowl and Manning's restaurant buildings. Those vernacular-architecture classics were razed for apartment behemoths, which at this writing haven't been built yet. At the southeast corner of 15th and Market you can take a #15 bus back to your start.

CONNECTING THE WALKS

This walk connects easily to two other walks. At 24th Ave. NW and NW Market St. you're a half mile east of the end of Walk 10. At 14th Ave. NW and NW 46th St. you're a half mile northwest of Walk 14 at the Burke-Gilman Trail and NW 43rd St.

POINTS OF INTEREST

Galway Traders galwaytraders.com, 7518 15th Ave. NW, 206-784-9343

Scandinavian Specialties scanspecialties.com, 6719 15th Ave. NW, 206-784-7020

Zesto's Burger and Fish House zestosseatle.com, 6416 15th Ave. NW, 206-783-3350

St. Alphonsus Parish stalphonsus-sea.org, 5816 15th Ave. NW, 206-784-6464

The RE Store re-store.org, 1440 NW 52nd St., 206-297-9119

Mars Hill Church marshillchurch.org, 1401 NW Leary Way, 206-816-3500

Mike's Chili Parlor Tavern mikeschiliparlor.com, 1447 NW Ballard Way, 206-782-4641

Tractor Tavern tractortavern.com, 5213 Ballard Ave. NW, 206-789-3599

Sunset Tavern sunsettavern.com, 5433 Ballard Ave. NW, 206-784-4880

Leif Erikson Lodge leiferiksonlodge.com, 2245 NW 57th St., 206-783-1274

route summary

1. Start at 15th Ave. NW and NW 75th St., walking south.

2. Turn east on NW 52nd St.

3. Turn south on 14th Ave. NW.

4. Turn west on NW 46th St. back toward 15th.

5. Turn north on 15th.

6. Turn west on NW Leary Way.

7. Dogleg south on 17th Ave. NW to NW 48th St.

8. Turn west on 48th.

9. Turn northwest on Ballard Ave. NW.

10. Turn west on NW Market St.

11. Go north on 24th Ave. NW.

12. Turn east on NW 57th St.

13. Just east of Leif Erickson Lodge on 57th, turn south and cut through a parking lot to NW 56th St.

14. Cross a midblock crosswalk at 56th; cut through another parking lot to the Ballard Square building.

15. Descend the interior stairs to Ballard Square's main floor; exit the building's south side back onto Market.

16. Walk east on Market back to 15th Ave. NW.

Ballard Firehouse

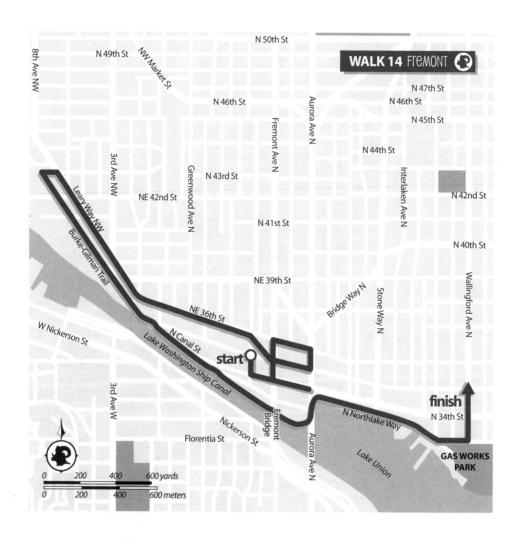

N 50th St

8th Ave NW

N 49th St

NW Market St

N 47th St

N 46th St

Aurora Ave N

N 46th St

N 45th St

Fremont Ave N

N 44th St

3rd Ave NW

Greenwood Ave N

N 43rd St

Interlaken Ave N

N 42nd St

NE 42nd St

N 41st St

Leary Way NW

N 40th St

Burke-Gilman Trail

NE 39th St

Bridge Way N

Stone Way N

Wallingford Ave N

NE 36th St

W Nickerson St

N Canal St

Lake Washington Ship Canal

start

3rd Ave W

N Northlake Way

finish
N 34th St

Florentia St

Nickerson St

Fremont Bridge

Aurora Ave N

Lake Union

GAS WORKS PARK

0   200   400   600 yards
0   200   400   600 meters

14 Fremont: Center of at Least One Universe

BOUNDARIES: **N. 43rd St., N. Canal St., N. Northlake Way, and Wallingford Ave. N.**
DISTANCE: **3¾ miles**
DIFFICULTY: **Moderate (brief inclines at the beginning and end)**
PARKING: **Metered street parking**
PUBLIC TRANSIT: **Metro routes #26, 28, 30, and 31 stop at Fremont Ave. N. and N. 34th St.**

A once-separate mill town annexed to Seattle, Fremont fell into a long decline after 1932, when the Aurora Bridge diverted traffic away from the neighborhood. It became a hangout for fringe populations. Those subcultures eventually included collegiate hippies, who brought funky shops and arts studios to the neighborhood. More recently, it's become a nightlife and dining destination, promoting itself as the "Center of the Universe." Its most famous attraction is the annual Solstice Parade, with artsy floats, alternative marching bands, and body-painted bicyclists. Even during the rest of the year, Fremont prides itself on doing things with a little more eccentricity and a little more flair, as you're about to see.

● **Start under the Fremont Rocket at N. 35th St. and Evanston Ave. N. This 55-foot-tall space-age decorative sign used to adorn a now-demolished surplus store in Belltown (Walk 5). It stands atop two of Fremont's several art and fashion boutiques, Burnt Sugar and Frankie. Turn south one block on Evanston, past the T-shirt store Destee Nation.**

● **Turn east onto the north side of N. 34th St. Behind you is the Red Door Alehouse, highlighted by a replica of the red "R" sign that once stood atop the Rainier brewery in SoDo. To your left at Fremont Ave. N. is the neighborhood's main shopping drag (which we'll track back to). To your right is the Fremont Bridge. The neighborhood's chief icon was built (along with the Lake Washington Ship Canal it crosses) in 1917. It's one of the busiest drawbridges in the United States, rising an average of 35 times a day.**

● **Cross Fremont Ave., then cross 34th. At a traffic island in this crossing you meet** *Waiting for the Interurban,* **Richard Beyer's 1979 aluminum sculpture commemorating the long-gone streetcar line that ran up Fremont Ave. It depicts five people and a dog** standing beneath a shelter; the dog's face resembles community organizer Arman Stepanian. You might see decor and fashion accessories added to the figures by citizens to denote special occasions.

- Cross to the south side of 34th and walk east, past one of the office parks that replaced the lumber mills. Halfway down this long block you find a latter-day sequel sculpture, *Late for the Interurban*. It depicts J. P. Patches and Gertrude, clown stars of a legendary local kids' TV show that ran from 1958 to 1981.

- When you reach the underside of the Aurora Bridge, cross 34th. At 34th and Troll Ave. (the short street under the tall bridge) is History House, a neighborhood cultural facility with a covered sculpture garden in front. From there turn back to Fremont Ave.

- Turn north onto Fremont Ave., past quaint old shop buildings (and modern "mixed-use" buildings trying to fit in), housing Greek, Thai, and sushi restaurants and merchants selling hammered dulcimers, designer shoes, and vinyl records.

- At N. 36th St. (with the Dubliner and Dad Watson's bars), turn east and uphill, past the Fremont Baptist Church's blocky-brick solidity, to the Fremont Troll. The 1990 concrete sculpture, commissioned from four local artists, was built to turn the vacant land under the Aurora Bridge from blight to tourist attraction. The whole thing's 16 feet tall; the troll's one eye is a hubcap; the car in its paw is a real VW Beetle.

- Turn south on Troll Ave. to N. 35th St.; turn west onto the south side of 35th, past an elegant Spanish mission–style Seattle Public Library branch. Beyond it is a new pocket park with a circular walkway. Beyond that is the intimate 35th Street Bistro. Beyond that, enjoy artist Parris Broderick's cartoony 1991 mural advertising the bistro's defunct predecessor, Still Life in Fremont.

- You're now at the five-way intersection of 35th, Fremont Ave., and Fremont Pl. N. Cross to the west side of Fremont Ave. to the well-curated Fremont Place Book Company. Take a right across 35th to the north side of Fremont Pl. Turn northwest, past a triangular building containing the Bliss fashion store and Espresso To Go (the most ornate tiny coffee stand you'll see anywhere).

Across an alley, the exquisite vintage shop Deluxe Junk occupies the lower level of a Masonic lodge. Beyond that stands a 16-foot bronze sculpture of Vladimir Lenin. A local collector acquired this monument of strident kitsch from a Slovakian scrap yard in 1993, literally rescuing it from the trash heap of history.

- Fremont Pl. bends west-northwest and becomes N. 36th St. To your right, the sedate grounds of a funeral home belie the noisy place this street can be after sundown. To your left, the reclaimed neon sign of a '50s bathing beauty marks High Dive, the first of the street's live music clubs.

- Continue on 36th beyond Dayton Ave. N. On your right, a former supermarket holds Roxy's Diner (originally a deli specializing in NY-style sandwiches, now grown to a full-service restaurant with a speakeasy-esque bar in the back). West of this are Ballroom (a swank bar and pool hall) and a Caffe Ladro coffeehouse. On the left side, Fremont Coffee Company occupies an entire historic bungalow.

On the north side of 36th beyond Francis Ave. N., Nectar is a music club with a covered outdoor patio. West of Phinney Ave. N. are several pubs, anchored by the George and Dragon, that cater to hardcore soccer fans. All are regularly packed during Sounders FC matches.

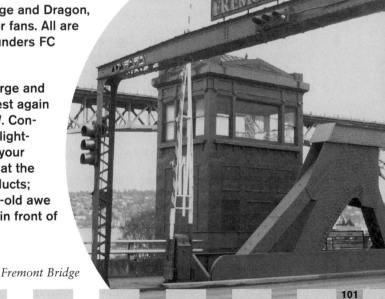

- Two blocks beyond the George and Dragon, 36th bends northwest again and becomes Leary Way NW. Continue as Leary segues from light-industrial to residential. Let your inner eight-year-old snicker at the sign for Tacoma Screw Products; then let your inner four-year-old awe at the life-size bear statues in front of

Fremont Bridge

the Brown Bear Car Wash. Souls of all ages will enjoy the small yard of rescued neon signs at Leary and 6th Ave. NW.

At 4320 Leary, an unmarked triangular 1920s building houses a recording studio that's had many names and owners since 1978. The first Nirvana and Soundgarden albums, among hundreds of others, were made there.

● Take a left onto NW 43rd St., along the south side of the Hale's Ales brewery and pub. Its back warehouse is seasonally used as a performance space. At its circus-decor entrance take a left onto the Burke-Gilman Trail, a former rail right-of-way that's become a popular walking, jogging, and biking path. Your first blocks along the Burke-Gilman abut warehouses, rail sidings, and a cement plant. Shrubbery and small trees have been added along the trail's sides to make it look at least a little green.

Once the trail parallels the north side of the Ship Canal, you're among wide lawns with a variety of trees, hugging the water. You can spot ducks, kayaks, and yachts. At Phinney Ave. N., the park sports two wire-frame dinosaurs (built for a Pacific Science Center exhibit), increasingly covered in topiary ivy. Also here, you can take a one-block detour left on Phinney to Theo Chocolates or Brouwer's Cafe (a Belgian-style pub).

● Continue or resume along the Burke-Gilman. To your left are the office-park buildings built where Fremont's sawmills had been. The trail bends under the Fremont Bridge, then curves north into park space under the Aurora Bridge's pillars. It then bends inland from the Ship Canal.

● At Stone Way N. take a short right-left dogleg closer to the water, along the walking and biking lane of N. Northlake Way. You see some marinas and the Lake Deli-Mart (a classic corrugated-steel Quonset hut).

● Continue on Northlake to Gas Works Park. This green jewel on Lake Union's northern crown was reclaimed in the 1970s from a coal gasification plant, rendered surplus when natural-gas pipelines reached the Pacific Northwest. A few pieces of the plant have been preserved as industrial sculpture within the park, which is otherwise given to open spaces and picnic tables.

● From here you can backtrack to the Fremont retail core. Alternately, climb an outdoor staircase connecting Northlake with Wallingford Ave. N. From the top of the steps, walk uphill on Wallingford. At Wallingford and N. 34th St. is the 200-foot-long headquarters of Avtech, an aerospace-electronics maker. The building looked more homey when it had a big neon sign on its roof for its original occupant, Grandma's Cookies. At the northwest corner of Wallingford and N. 35th St. is a #26 bus stop, leading back to Fremont Ave.

CONNECTING THE WALKS

This walk connects easily to four other walks. At N. 36th and Fremont you're a half mile south of Walk 17. At 36th and Troll you're a half mile south-southeast of Walk 15. At the Burke-Gilman Trail and 43rd you're a half mile southeast of Walk 13. At Northlake and Wallingford you're three-quarters of a mile west of Walk 19.

POINTS OF INTEREST

Fremont Rocket and Burnt Sugar and Frankie Boutiques store.burntsugarfrankie.com, 601 N. 35th St., 206-545-0699

History House historyhouse.org, 709 N. 34th St., 206-675-8875

Seattle Public Library, Fremont Branch spl.org, 731 N. 35th St.

High Dive highdiveseattle.com, 513 N. 36th St., 206-632-9212

Fremont Coffee Company fremontcoffee.net, 459 N. 36th St., 206-632-3633

Nectar nectarlounge.com, 412 N. 36th St., 206-632-2020

George & Dragon Pub georgeanddragonpub.com, 206 N. 36th St, 206-545-6864

Hale's Ales Pub halesbrewery.com, 4301 Leary Way NW, 206-706-1544

Fremont Bridge seattle.gov/transportation/bridges, Fremont Ave. N. south of N. Northlake Way

Gas Works Park seattle.gov/parks, 2101 N. Northlake Way

route summary

1. Start on Evanston Ave. N., walking south from N. 35th St.

2. Turn east on N. 34th St. two blocks to Troll Ave. N.

3. Cross and backtrack on 34th.

4. Turn north on Fremont Ave. N.

5. Turn east on N. 36th St.

6. Turn south on Troll Ave.

7. Turn west on N. 35th St.

8. Take a diagonal right onto Fremont Pl. N., which becomes N. 36th St and later Leary Way NW.

9. Turn left on NW 43rd St.

10. Turn southeast on the Burke-Gilman Trail.

11. Turn southeast on N. Northlake Way, to Wallingford Ave. N.

12. Either backtrack west on Northlake, or walk north to Wallingford and N. 35th St. and take a #26 bus back to Fremont Ave.

Lenin statue

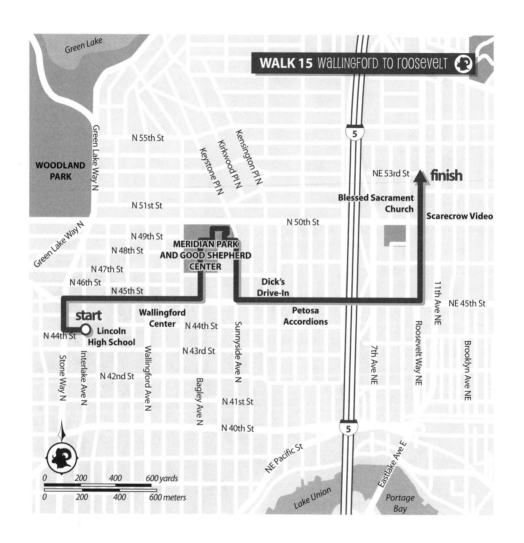

WALK 15 Wallingford to Roosevelt

15 Wallingford to Roosevelt: Bizarre Gifts to Obscure Flicks

BOUNDARIES: **N. 44th St., Stone Way N., NE 53rd St., and Roosevelt Way NE**
DISTANCE: **2¼ miles**
DIFFICULTY: **Easy (two slight inclines)**
PARKING: **Limited free street parking**
PUBLIC TRANSIT: **Metro routes #16 and 44 stop near the walk's start at N. 45th St. and Stone Way N.**

Unlike the founders of Ballard and Fremont, John Wallingford wasn't an industrialist. He was a real estate dealer. He and his fellow developers platted a "streetcar suburb" between Lake Union and Green Lake. It became a bedroom community with one of the strongest concentrations of Craftsman bungalows (early Seattle's favorite home style). Here, families drawn by Lake Union's industry mingled with the University of Washington community. Later, Wallingford became a stronghold of aging hippies; you're still more likely to spot a gray male ponytail here than anywhere in town, and one store specializes in selling buttons and bumper stickers adorned with lefty political slogans. Another store specializes in "messages" of a more playful sort. It's one of your first stops on this walk. One of your last stops will be a video store where you can get DVDs filmed in one language, dubbed in another, and subtitled in a third (none of them English).

● **Start in front of Lincoln High School, N. 44th St. and Interlake Ave. N.** The Edwardian brick edifice was a regular high school from 1907 to 1981. By the late 1980s it was depicted as a gang-ridden wasteland in the horror film *Class of 1999*. The school district now uses it as an interim replacement for schools whose own buildings are being remodeled.

● **Go west one block on 44th to Stone Way N.** by a big hardware store. Head north two blocks on Stone to N. 45th St. Three of the corners on this intersection hold big recent mixed-use buildings. But you're headed to the oldest building here, a former state liquor store at the northeast corner. You won't miss its bright red-and-yellow paint job, or the friendly monsters painted on top of that. This is Archie McPhee, a gift, toy, and souvenir store unlike any other. Tofu mints! Nacho lip balm! Gummy bacon! Plastic pickles emitting yodeling noises! Dashboard Jesus dolls! Inflatable toast! A "Crazy Cat Lady" action figure! Stuffed latex vultures! You might want to linger for hours, but you've got places to go.

● Walk east along the north side of 45th. Beyond Interlake Ave. N. is the Alphabet Soup children's bookstore, one of several storefronts on this street inside classic Craftsman bungalows. Beyond Woodlawn Ave. N. stands Sun Cleaners' bright sunburst sign. Two buildings away, the May Thai restaurant was designed to look like an ornate suburban Thai house. At Densmore Ave. N., the 45th Street Community Clinic occupies a comely, two-story old fire station. Kitty-corner from there, a Spanish-style row of storefronts includes great beer and wine stores.

Continue on the north side of 45th past Wallingford Ave. N., where two-story QFC supermarket bears some non-chain-standard signage, giant neon block letters spelling WALLINGFORD. In 2000, QFC was buying neighborhood stores around town, including this site's prior occupant, Food Giant. Neighborhood activists demanded the new owners keep the FOOD GIANT sign, a local landmark since the 1950s. This compromise incorporates seven of the old sign's nine letters. Across at the southeast corner of 45th and Wallingford, a big wood elementary school was revamped in the '80s into the Wallingford Center mall.

Beyond Burke Ave. N., Not A Number Cards and Gifts is like Archie McPhee for the political set, with anti-car-culture bumper stickers and antimaterialism merchandise. It's next to Teahouse Kuan Yin, selling gourmet loose leaf teas, and across from Murphy's, a neighborhood Irish bar. Beyond Meridian Ave. N., the plain stucco facade of Moon Temple hides a venerable neighborhood Chinese restaurant and bar. Across from it are the two Guild 45th Theater buildings. The eastern building is the original, a legendary art-house cinema for more than 50 years. Between it and the newer Guild 45th II is the Wallingford Pizza House, serving Chicago-style pizza out of a 1913 bungalow.

● Turn north on Bagley Ave. N., a narrow residential street. Just beyond N. 46th St., there's a dead end for drivers; keep walking into Meridian Park. It's the former grounds of a Catholic girls' home, the Home of the Good Shepherd (1906–1973). Here on the grounds' back side are a playground (with sculptures depicting children's-book characters), an apple orchard, gardens, and a P-Patch community garden.

The home's manor house–style main building looms to your right. It's now the Good Shepherd Center, run by preservation group Historic Seattle. Its vast square footage includes a performance space (in the former chapel), artist and senior housing units, community-group offices, a yoga center, and a private K–5 school.

- Take a right turn around the north side of the Good Shepherd Center, then another right toward the massive edifice's east entrance. Take a left down its front promenade, out of the grounds and onto Sunnyside Ave. N. Turn right (south) on Sunnyside. At N. 46th St. is the small, classy Elim Baptist Church. At 45th and Sunnyside, the Erotic Bakery offers its own flavor of iconography.

- Resume walking east on 45th. Open Books, an all-poetry bookstore, occupies the attached garage of an old house just beyond Sunnyside. Beyond 1st Ave. NE, the original Dick's Drive-In has supplied great cheap burgers and fries since 1954. Across from it on 2nd Ave. NE, Golden Oldies Records ("Open Eight Days a Week") is a trove of collectible vinyl; its wall now bears a hippie-esque mural depicting Jimi Hendrix, Kurt Cobain, and other rock icons.

East of Thackeray Pl. NE, the Hawai'i General Store and Gallery offers both authentic and tourist-culture gifts and foods from the islands. Near 4th Ave. NE, the jet-black storefront of Petosa Accordions gives a deceptively modernist front to a shop that's made handcrafted squeezeboxes since 1922. The sales room includes a display of more than 140 historic instruments.

Continue on the north side of what's now NE 45th St., across the Interstate 5 overpass. Just beyond 7th Ave. NE, the Seattle Go Center teaches the Japanese board game as a metaphor for life. Just east of there, turn your internal clock back to 1971 at the Blue Moon Tavern, Seattle's venerable literary-hippie dive bar. At 9th Ave. NE, the Metro Cinemas tenplex anchors a retail complex on the former site of a Chevrolet dealership. The ex-Chevy showroom, at 45th and Roosevelt Way NE, now houses a bicycle shop.

- Turn north along the west side of Roosevelt Way. At NE 50th St., the Seven Gables Theater is an intimate, elegant film palace. As local film insiders know, the building has only six gables. These insiders also gather at Cinema Books, a bookseller in the same building with new and old tomes about new and old films. Across 50th, the

Seattle Public Library's University Branch is an always-welcome instance of a stock Carnegie-funded library design. Cross to Roosevelt's east side and continue north to Scarecrow Video. Claiming nearly 100,000 titles in stock (including many foreign films unreleased in this country), it's been called the best video store in the United States.

● Walking on Roosevelt toward NE 53rd St., to your left is the Blessed Sacrament Catholic Church's imposing spire. To your right are German-style and New York–style delis. To return to your start, backtrack south on Roosevelt to 45th and take a #44 bus to Stone Way.

CONNECTING THE WALKS

This walk connects easily to four other walks. It starts a half mile north of Walk 14 and ends a quarter mile south of Walk 18. At 50th and Roosevelt you're four blocks west of Walk 19. At the Good Shepherd Center you're three-quarters of a mile south of Walk 16.

POINTS OF INTEREST

Archie McPhee archiemcpheeseattle.com, 1300 N. 45th St., 206-297-0240
Not A Number Cards and Gifts notanumbergifts.com, 1905 N. 45th St., 206-784-0965
Good Shepherd Center historicseattle.org/projects/gsc.aspx, 4649 Sunnyside Ave. N
Dick's Drive-In dicksdrivein.com, 111 NE 45th St., 206-634-0300
Petosa Accordions petosa.com, 313 NE 45th St., 206-632-2700
Blue Moon Tavern bluemoonseattle.wordpress.com, 712 NE 45th St., 206-675-9116
Cinema Books cinemabooks.net, 4753 Roosevelt Way NE, 206-547-7667
Scarecrow Video scarecrow.com, 5030 Roosevelt Way NE, 206-524-8554
Blessed Sacrament Church blessed-sacrament.org, 5041 9th Ave. NE, 206-546-3020

route summary

1. Start on N. 44th St., walking west from Interlake Ave. N.

2. Turn north on Stone Way N.

3. Turn east on N. 45th St.

4. Turn north on Bagley Ave. N. into Meridian Playground.

5. Walk around the north and east sides of the Good Shepherd Center.

6. Turn south on Sunnyside Ave. N.

7. Resume walking east on N. 45th.

8. Turn north on Roosevelt Way NE, to NE 53rd St.

9. To return to your start, backtrack south on Roosevelt to 45th and take a #44 bus to Stone Way.

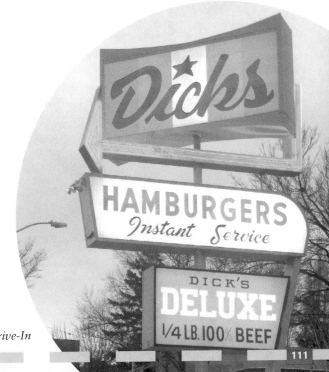

The original Dick's Drive-In

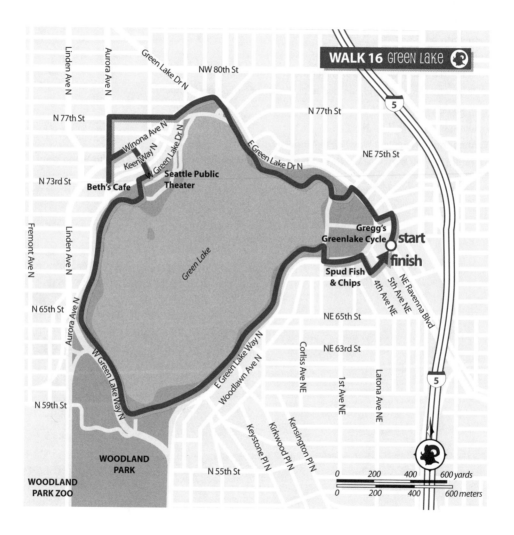

Linden Ave N

Aurora Ave N

Green Lake Dr N

NW 80th St

N 77th St

N 77th St

Winona Ave N

Keen Way N

N Green Lake Dr N

E Green Lake Dr N

NE 75th St

N 73rd St

Beth's Cafe

Seattle Public Theater

Fremont Ave N

Linden Ave N

Aurora Ave N

Green Lake

Gregg's Greenlake Cycle

start

finish

Spud Fish & Chips

NE Ravenna Blvd

5th Ave NE

4th Ave NE

N 65th St

E Green Lake Way N

NE 65th St

NE 63rd St

Corliss Ave NE

1st Ave NE

Latona Ave NE

W Green Lake Way N

Woodlawn Ave N

N 59th St

Kensington Pl N

Kirkwood Pl N

Keystone Pl N

WOODLAND PARK

N 55th St

WOODLAND PARK ZOO

5

5

0   200   400   600 yards

0   200   400   600 meters

16 Green Lake: Beware of Manic Joggers

BOUNDARIES: **NE Ravenna Blvd., E. Green Lake Way N., N. 77th St., and Aurora Ave. N.**
DISTANCE: **4 miles**
DIFFICULTY: **Easy (essentially all flat)**
PARKING: **Metered street parking along Woodlawn**
PUBLIC TRANSIT: **Metro routes #16, 26, and 48 stop at this walk's start.**

A big spot of water and open space surrounded by North Seattle's residential calm, Green Lake got its name simply because an early surveyor noted how green it was, because of algae gathering along its shallow bottom. The lake got even greener when city officials made it even shallower. Later officials have tried to make the lake less green over the years by cracking down on algae and aquatic plants, with mixed success. Through all this time, the 3-mile path around the lake's perimeter has remained a popular spot for seeing and being seen, for running, jogging, bicycling, roller skating, canoeing, swimming, and just plain walking.

- Start at the southeast corner of NE Ravenna Blvd. and Woodlawn Ave. NE, in the east Green Lake business district. Ravenna is one of the wide boulevard streets platted by the Olmsted Brothers in 1903, running for 20 miles and connecting most of the city's major parks (Walk 24). This boulevard follows, more or less, the route of the old Ravenna Creek, which used to drain Green Lake's water into Lake Washington. To your left on Woodlawn, Gregg's Greenlake Cycle occupies an old building with a Spanish colonial–inspired roof. To your right is a new mixed-use complex.

- Head northeast on Woodlawn past NE 71st St. On your left is Little Red Hen, a home for live country entertainment. Its food is as down-home as its music; there's nothing like walking the lake on a tummy full of biscuits, bacon, and gravy.

- Turn west on the north side of NE 72nd St. past a Nautilus gym, My Place Cafe (a little breakfast place), and the Green Lake Bar and Grill. Turn right onto East Green Lake Dr. N., walking northwest for three blocks, past the Seattle Public Library's stately Green Lake Branch (a twin to the equally stately University Branch, in Walk 15).

● Turn left at East Green Lake and Latona Ave. NE, onto a sidewalk beside a driveway leading into Green Lake Park. The park lies mostly on land reclaimed when the lake was lowered by seven feet in 1911, as recommended in the Olmsted Brothers' city-wide park plan. It's a place of active leisure, particularly this part of it. To your left is the Green Lake Community Center, with a heavily used indoor pool and gym. That's surrounded by a playground, a boat-rental shop, tennis courts, and soccer and soft-ball fields. Walk west on this sidewalk toward the lake.

● Take a right turn onto the paved Green Lake Path, which curves around the lake for 3.5 miles. The inside lane of the two-lane path is reserved for walkers and runners. Bicyclists and roller-skaters are restricted to the one-way outside lane. If you're here on a summer weekend afternoon, you'll soon learn why; traffic levels can make this path seem like a nonmotorized freeway, with sunbathers and hyperactive children as roadside distractions.

● Just before you approach a small wading pool, you see a side path heading right. Turn onto this side path, out of the park and back onto East Green Lake Dr. heading west. There's a small restaurant row here.

Continue heading west on what becomes West Green Lake Dr. N. past two intersections, then take a soft right onto Winona Ave. N. Then immediately take another soft right onto N. 77th St. for two blocks to Aurora Ave. N., part of the old Pacific Coast Highway. It's a bold-as-brass slice of the old boisterous roadside America.

● Turn south on Aurora's west side, past gaudy storefronts offering motorcycles, used computers, guns, and lawn mowers, as well as a couple of bars specializing in imported beers. Just north of N. 73rd St. is Aurora's heart and soul, Beth's Cafe. Since 1954, this unreconstructed diner has served hearty portions, including the specialty 12-egg omelets, 24 hours a day.

● Backtrack up Aurora and cross at the first stoplight onto Winona Ave. N., going east. If Beth's didn't entice your appetite, you can pick up something at the PCC Natural Market here. Continue east on Winona one block to Stone Ave. N.

- Turn southeast on Stone three blocks back to West Green Lake Dr. You're at the parking entrance to the Seattle Public Theater, a gorgeous 1916 bathhouse used for stage shows since the 1970s. Walk south back into Green Lake Park.

- Rejoin the Green Lake Path, walking around the lake's west side. At the lake's southwest corner, a preserved segment of concrete grandstand seating marks the former site of the Aqua Theater, where plays and "Aqua Follies" musicals were held in the '50s and '60s. It's now the Green Lake Small Craft Center, home to youth rowing and canoeing programs.

- Follow the path as it bends east, past the Pitch and Putt Golf Course, then curves northeast. As you approach the softball fields you find a south turn out of the park, back onto East Green Lake Dr. N.

- Go east on East Green Lake for three blocks, to 4th Ave. NE and Spud Fish & Chips.

- Go southeast on 4th one block, back to Woodlawn. Turn northeast on Woodlawn for two blocks, back to your start at Ravenna.

CONNECTING THE WALKS

This walk connects easily to two other walks. It starts a half mile northwest of Walk 18. On Aurora, you're a steep half mile east of Walk 17.

POINTS OF INTEREST

Gregg's Greenlake Cycle greggscycles.com, 7007 Woodlawn Ave. NE, 206-523-1822

Little Red Hen littleredhen.com, 7115 Woodlawn Ave. NE, 206-522-1168

Green Lake Community Center seattle.gov/parks/centers/grnlakcc.htm, 7201 East Green Lake Dr. N., 206-684-0780

Beth's Cafe bethscafe.com, 7311 Aurora Ave. N., 206-782-5588

Seattle Public Theater seattlepublictheater.org, 7312 West Green Lake Dr. N., 206-524-1300

Spud Fish & Chips spudfishandchips.com, 6860 East Green Lake Dr. N., 206-524-0565

route summary

1. Start on Woodlawn Ave. NE, walking northeast from NE Ravenna Blvd.
2. Turn west on NE 72nd St.
3. Turn northwest on East Green Lake Dr. N.
4. Turn southeast on Latona Ave. NE into Green Lake Park.
5. Turn right onto the Green Lake Path, which curves from north to northwest.
6. Make a right turn at the wading pool, back to East Green Lake Dr.
7. Take a soft right onto Winona Ave. N. Take another soft right onto N. 77th St.
8. Turn south on Aurora Ave. N.'s west side, to N. 73rd St.
9. Backtrack to Aurora and Winona; turn east on Winona.
10. Turn southeast on Stone Ave. N. back to Green Lake Park.
11. Reenter the park and rejoin the Green Lake Path, walking southwest, then curving east and northeast.
12. At the softball fields, turn south out of the park.
13. Turn east on East Green Lake Dr. N.
14. Go southeast on 4th Ave. NE.
15. Turn northeast on Woodlawn two blocks back to your start.

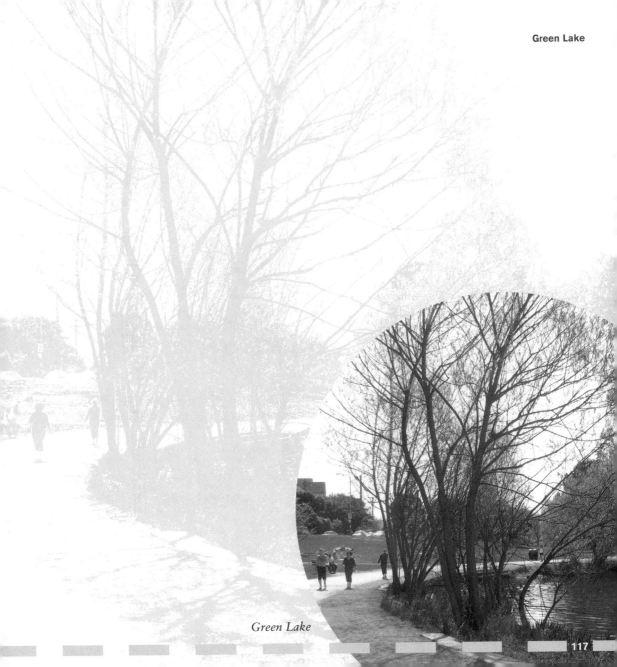

Green Lake

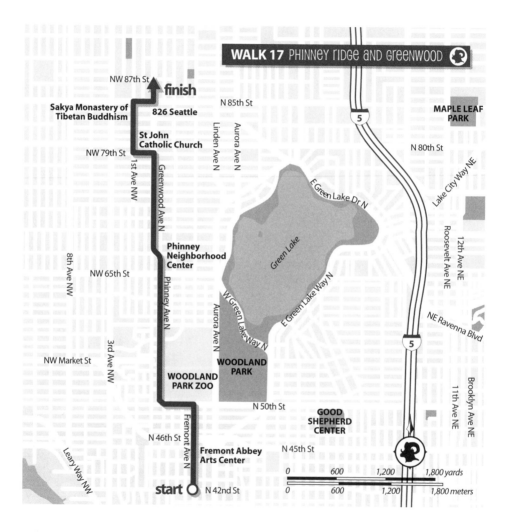

WALK 17 PHINNEY RIDGE AND GREENWOOD

NW 87th St

finish

Sakya Monastery of
Tibetan Buddhism

826 Seattle

N 85th St

St John
Catholic Church

NW 79th St

Linden Ave N

Aurora Ave N

5

MAPLE LEAF
PARK

N 80th St

1st Ave NW

Greenwood Ave N

E Green Lake Dr N

Lake City Way NE

Green Lake

12th Ave NE

Roosevelt Ave NE

Phinney
Neighborhood
Center

8th Ave NW

NW 65th St

Phinney Ave N

W Green Lake Way N

E Green Lake Way N

5

NE Ravenna Blvd

3rd Ave NW

NW Market St

Aurora Ave N

WOODLAND
PARK

11th Ave NE

Brooklyn Ave NE

WOODLAND
PARK ZOO

N 50th St

GOOD
SHEPHERD
CENTER

Leary Way NW

Fremont Ave N

N 46th St

Fremont Abbey
Arts Center

N 45th St

| 0 | 600 | 1,200 | 1,800 yards |
| 0 | 600 | 1,200 | 1,800 meters |

start N 42nd St

17 PHINNEY RIDGE AND GREENWOOD: THE ZOO AND OTHER WELL-MAINTAINED HABITATS

BOUNDARIES: **N. 42nd St., Fremont Ave. N., 1st Ave. NW, and N. 87th St.**
DISTANCE: **3 miles**
DIFFICULTY: **Moderate (one short incline at the start)**
PARKING: **Free street parking along Fremont Ave. N. and surrounding streets; $5 parking in Woodland Park south lot**
PUBLIC TRANSIT: **Metro route #5 stops at this walk's start.**

Phinney Ridge is North Seattle's topographic "spine," rising for two miles between the traditionally industrial Ballard and Fremont and the traditionally more bourgeois northeast neighborhoods. At the ridge's peak stands the Woodland Park Zoo, a crossroads of species as well as cultures. It's a worldwide leader in showcasing its various critters within naturalistic habitat displays. Before and after passing the zoo, this walk takes you through some neighborhood business blocks that have gradually become more boutique-y in recent years.

● Start at N. 42nd St. and Fremont Ave. N., near the former Buckaroo Tavern's frontier-style 1908 wood building. It's the start of a cozy little business district, which includes some fine dining spots, a major musical instrument store, and a jam-packed deli-mart. Its newest *and* oldest attraction is the Fremont Abbey Arts Center, a performance and workshop space in a 1914 brick church building.

● Walk north on Fremont to N. 50th St., the south border of Woodland Park. The 92-acre park was originally the private estate of developer Guy Phinney. The city bought the land from his widow, then developed it according to the Olmsted Brothers' citywide park plan, with the zoo as its centerpiece. The zoo's side entrance is here. So are a few free parking spaces outside the zoo's gates. Of particular note is the exquisitely landscaped rose garden east of the zoo entrance, with two white fountains and an art deco relief mural.

● Turn west along the park's south side, past an oversize bronze statue of a Spanish-American War soldier, to Phinney Ave N. Turn north along Phinney's east side, past the zoo's main entrance. Woodland Park is one of the nation's most renowned zoo-logical parks, a leader in "immersion" exhibits that simulate animals' natural habitats. It's also a great walking site in its own right. But for this walk continue along Phinney. Woodland Park's northwest corner, at Phinney and N. 59th St., is another public open space outside the zoo's fences.

Continue north along Phinney, into a neighborhood business strip flourishing with gift boutiques, small apparel shops, and cool eating and drinking spots. The latter catego-ry's grande dame is Sully's Snowgoose Saloon (formerly La Boheme), at Phinney and N. 62nd St. The Repeal-era tavern looks like a Tudor cottage on the outside and a ski lodge on the inside. Another neighborhood favorite is Mae's Phinney Ridge Cafe, an adorably kitschy breakfast spot near N. 65th St. A block north of that is the Phinney Neighborhood Center, an arts and community-meeting space in a preserved wooden schoolhouse.

● At N. 67th St., follow the arterial as it doglegs into Greenwood Ave. N. Along the north end of this curving transitional segment is Red Mill Burgers, whose hearty handmade fare attracts long lines on weekend afternoons. Just beyond the S-curve on Green-wood's west side, the Francine Seders Gallery is a treasury of Northwest contempo-rary art.

● Continue north on Greenwood, a pleasant stroll alongside more nice shops and eateries. The latter range from El Chupacabra's creative Mexican fare to the Stum-bling Goat Bistro's organic gourmet menu. The former include stores selling clothes by local designers, shoes, pianos, antiques, rugs, knitting supplies, toys, pet sup-plies, greeting cards, picture frames, and baked goods. Then there's a business best described as "only in Seattle"—Espresso Dental, where you can get wide awake before you get numbed.

● At Greenwood and N. 79th St. turn west for one long block, to 1st Ave. NW and the stately, Romanesque edifice of St. John the Evangelist Catholic Church with its dome-topped square tower. Turn north on 1st to N. 83rd St. and a very different take on religious architecture at the Sakya Monastery of Tibetan Buddhism. It's a 1920s Pres-byterian church building that's been completely redone and repainted in the tradi-tional bright Tibetan colors. A large bell-shaped stupa (a sacred container with other sacred objects placed inside it) sits at its front. It's one of many holy objects from India, Tibet, and Nepal adorning the building inside and out.

- Continuing north on 1st you soon view the huge red sign for the Fred Meyer big-box store on N. 85th St., anchor of the main Greenwood business district. Turn east on 85th, through an old-fashioned main street district. On the south side of 85th is Squirrel's Buy/Sell, a storefront attic of kitschy collectibles. On the north side, a onetime neighborhood cinema now houses Taproot Theater, a mainstream Christian troupe staging drawing-room comedies and moral-choice dramas.

- Cross to the southeast corner of 85th and Greenwood. Just south of this corner, a busy, bizarre storefront proclaims itself to be GREENWOOD SPACE TRAVEL SUPPLY CO. and promises ROCKET PARKING ON ROOF. It's really 826 Seattle, part of a national circuit of reading and educational centers cofounded by author and publisher Dave Eggers. The fake sci-fi advertising is intended to enthrall kids with the power of words even before they step inside.

- Turn back north on Greenwood, north of 85th. You're now outside Seattle's pre-1954 city limits, and in a one-block nightlife mini-mecca. Your dinner-and-drink choices range from the unapologetically working-class (Baranof, the Crosswalk Tavern) to spiffy (Gainsbourg, Olive You), to handcrafted (Naked City Brewery & Alehouse, Wayward Coffeehouse). There's shopping too—used books, games, hobbies, and Mexican groceries.

- At the northwest corner of Greenwood and N. 87th St., you can take a #5 bus back to your starting point.

CONNECTING THE WALKS

This walk connects easily to three other walks. It starts a half mile north of Walk 14. At N. 46th St. and Fremont, you're a half mile west of Walk 15. At N. 77th St. and Greenwood Ave. N., you're a downhill half mile west of Walk 16.

POINTS OF INTEREST

Fremont Abbey Arts Center fremontabbey.org, 4272 Fremont Ave. N., 206-701-9270

Woodland Park Zoo zoo.org, 5500 Phinney Ave. N., 206-548-2500

Phinney Neighborhood Center phinneycenter.org, 6532 Phinney Ave. N., 206-783-2244

St. John the Evangelist Catholic Church stjohnsea.org, 121 N. 80th St., 206-782-2810

Sakya Monastery sakya.org, 108 NW 83rd St., 206-789-2573

826 Seattle 826seattle.org, 8414 Greenwood Ave. N., 206-725-2625

Baranof 8549 Greenwood Ave. N., 206-782-9260

route summary

1. Start on Fremont Ave. N., walking north from N. 42nd St.
2. Turn west on N. 50th St.
3. Turn north on Phinney Ave. N., which doglegs into Greenwood Ave. N.
4. Turn west on N. 79th St.
5. Turn north on 1st Ave. NW.
6. Turn east on N. 85th St.
7. Turn north on Greenwood, to N. 87th St.

Woodland Park rose garden

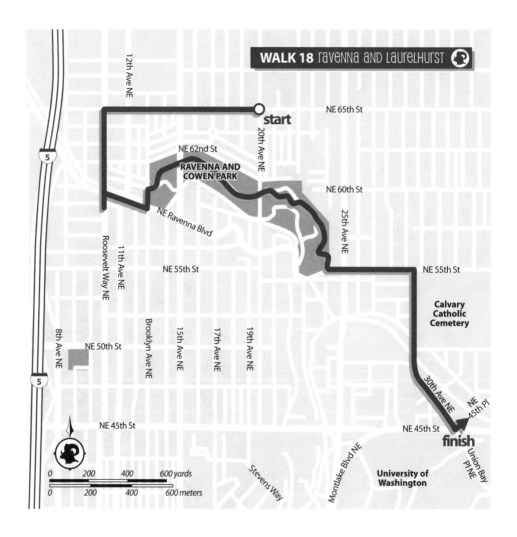

NE 65th St

start

NE 62nd St

RAVENNA AND
COWEN PARK

NE Ravenna Blvd

NE 60th St

NE 55th St

NE 55th St

12th Ave NE

20th Ave NE

25th Ave NE

Roosevelt Way NE

11th Ave NE

Brooklyn Ave NE

15th Ave NE

17th Ave NE

19th Ave NE

Calvary
Catholic
Cemetery

8th Ave NE

NE 50th St

30th Ave NE

NE PI

NE 45th St

NE 45th St

finish

Union Bay PI NE

Stevens Way

Montlake Blvd NE

University of
Washington

0   200   400   600 yards
0   200   400   600 meters

18 ravenna and Laurelhurst: creekside rambling

BOUNDARIES: **NE 65th St., NE 45th St., 30th Ave. NE, and Roosevelt Ave. NE**
DISTANCE: **3 miles**
DIFFICULTY: **Easy (two brief inclines)**
PARKING: **Free street parking along NE 65th St. and surrounding streets**
PUBLIC TRANSIT: **Metro route #71 stops at this walk's start.**

When you're in parts of Ravenna and Cowen Park, you can pretend you've stepped back in time, to when Seattle was still a tree-covered wilderness. The park's a second-growth forest; the original trees had been cut down by the 1920s. But after more than eight decades, these replacement trees have become tall, mature specimens in their own right. The park's especially grand when you're walking along the bottom of an old glacial ravine, where the developed city disappears from sight. The park's surrounding residential neighborhoods, traditionally home to University of Washington faculty members and other professionals, sport their own kind of spectacles, particularly at Christmastime.

- **Start on the north side of NE 65th St. at 20th Ave. NE, in front of Third Place Books. A well-stocked independent lit emporium, it's also got a skylit cafe and a basement pub. Across 20th, Gasoline Alley Antiques is a tiny storefront crammed to the ceiling with toys, buttons, and mementos invoking several generations' childhoods.**

- **Walk west on 65th. For the first few blocks, you're walking slightly uphill past classic Craftsman bungalows. At 15th Ave. NE you can see the stoic facade of Roosevelt High School, behind an ex-gas station now housing a produce stand. This street also marks the eastern boundary of the Roosevelt business district. On the left side of 65th beyond Brooklyn Ave. NE is the quaint pub and eatery Pies and Pints (that's pot pies, not dessert pies). On 65th's right side beyond 12th Ave. NE is the preserved deco storefront of Standard Records and Hi-Fi, a onetime classical LP store. This site is set to eventually become a light rail station.**

- **Turn south at 65th and Roosevelt Way NE, the heart of the Roosevelt strip. Rain City Burgers is at this intersection's northwest corner; Indonesian and East Indian food spots are nearby. Besides the usual neighborhood dining and shopping** opportunities, this strip has also attracted merchants selling two specific genres of goods—audio/video gear and New Age books and trinkets. Decorate your flat-screen home theater with Celtic rune stones!

Continue on Roosevelt south to NE 59th St. At this intersection's northeast corner, along the south wall of the Trading Musician music store, note the cute mural depicting an all-insect rock concert entitled "Larvae Live!" On the southeast corner there's Cafe Racer, an artists' hangout and watering hole. The front room features rotating exhibits by local artists. A side dining room holds a permanent kitsch painting collection called the "Official Bad Art Museum of Art."

● Backtrack north on Roosevelt one block, to NE Ravenna Blvd. As mentioned in Walk 16, this is one of the Olmsted plan boulevards, wide streets with grassy median strips crossing the city. Walk southeast on Ravenna for three blocks to Brooklyn Ave. NE; turn north on Brooklyn one block to Cowen Park's west entrance. Cowen is essentially a neighborhood playground area, immediately west of the more nature-oriented Ravenna Park. It's also got some quaint public art, such as little bronze statues of sea creatures and an oversize sundial within a grass circle.

● Take the main path curving northeast and downhill into the Ravenna Park Trail. Follow the half-mile main trail as it curves east, then southeast, through the bottom of the volcanic ravine alongside Ravenna Creek. At one point you're as much as 115 feet below the surrounding residential streets. At the trail's midpoint you walk under the Ravenna Park Bridge, a beautiful latticed-arch steel span that's now pedestrian-only. As you gently rise back toward street level, you see a stretch of Ravenna Creek that was "daylighted" in 2006; the water had previously been diverted through underground pipes.

● The park's southeast end is an open space facing NE 55th St., just west of 25th Ave. NE. From here you can walk north on 25th back to 65th St., then head west back to your start.

If you're walking this walk in December, take a brief detour east on 55th to Ravenna Ave. NE, then head north to NE Park Rd. The street annually becomes Candy Cane Lane, where every homeowner participates in elegant Christmas decorations.

SIDE TRIP: SAND POINT AND THE SOUND GARDEN

If you're up to it, continue beyond this walk's official end by rejoining the Burke-Gilman Trail at the old railroad trestle above NE 45th Pl., starting east then bending north. After 2 miles of walking past impressive postwar homes and peekaboo Lake Washington views, turn right at NE 70th St. Turn left at Sand Point Way NE, then right again at NE 74th St. You're in Warren G. Magnuson Park, created from a former naval airfield. These 350 lakeside acres include trails, picnic areas, an off-leash dog park, and preserved old brick Navy buildings.

Another part of the old airfield belongs to the National Oceanic and Atmospheric Administration. This campus (open to the public weekdays) includes a public art piece comprising mounted organ pipes that generate muted tones in the wind. It's the Sound Garden, namesake of the classic Seattle rock band.

● If you're continuing with this walk, turn east for a short uphill stretch on 55th. At the northeast corner of 55th and 25th is Kidd Valley, a venerable local family-dining spot. When it opened in the 1970s, its sign depicted a hippie chick in a halter top and cutoff jeans, leaning back on top of a giant hamburger. After citizen complaints, the image was replaced by something more abstract.

Just east of 55th and 28th Ave. NE is the Duchess Tavern, a UW student hangout dating back to the Repeal era. It's full of decor celebrating UW sports over the decades. At 30th Ave. NE, the Queen Mary Tea Room is a slice of old English propriety and quiet good taste.

● Turn south and downhill on 30th, a narrow tree-lined residential street, along the south side of Calvary Catholic Cemetery. At the intersection with Blakely Ave. NE, turn left to continue on 30th.

You soon see another intersection, with the Burke-Gilman Trail. If you can resist the temptation to join the jogging throngs crowding this stretch of the trail from sunup to sundown, continue on 30th past NE 49th St. That's the east entrance to the University Village mall. It contains a bevy of major upscale chain stores, ranging from Anthropologie to Zovo (a lingerie shop). It stands on what used to be the Seattle city dump, fictionalized as the setting for the local kids' TV show *J. P. Patches* (Walk 14).

- South of 49th, 30th Ave. curves southeast. It becomes Union Bay Place NE, an off-the-mall commercial strip where the storefronts are much more likely to be of the mom-and-pop variety. Union Bay Pl. ends at a five-way intersection with NE 45th St. and NE 45th Pl. In front of you are UW athletic fields. To your right is Burgermaster, another venerable family-dining spot. Taking a hard left onto 45th Pl., you see a short wooden railroad bridge, now part of the Burke-Gilman Trail.

- On the southeast side of 45th Pl., you can take a #65 bus to the University District and downtown. Or you can cut across the University Village lot to 25th Ave. NE and NE 47th St., in front of the Yves Delorme boutique. There you can take a #68 bus (which doesn't run Sundays or holidays) back to NE 65th St.

CONNECTING THE WALKS

This walk connects easily with three other walks. At NE Ravenna Blvd. you're a half mile north of Walks 15 and 19. At 65th and Roosevelt you're a half mile southeast of Walk 16.

POINTS OF INTEREST

Third Place Books ravenna.thirdplacebooks.com, 6504 20th Ave. NE, 206-736-5009

Gasoline Alley Antiques gasolinealleyantiques.com, 6501 20th Ave. NE, 206-524-1606

Trading Musician tradingmusician.com, 5908 Roosevelt Way NE, 206-522-6707

Cafe Racer caferacer.com, 5828 Roosevelt Way NE, 206-523-5282

Ravenna and Cowen Park seattle.gov/parks, 5849 15th Ave. NE, 206-548-2500

Calvary Catholic Cemetery acc-seattle.com/cemeteries/calvary.html, 5041 35th Ave. NE, 206-522-0996

University Village uvillage.com, 2673 NE University Village Way, 206-523-0622

route summary

1.   Start on NE 65th St. walking west from 20th Ave. NE.
2.   Turn south on Roosevelt Way NE to NE 59th St.
3.   Backtrack north to Roosevelt and NE Ravenna Blvd. Walk southeast on Ravenna.
4.   Turn north on Brooklyn Ave. NE to Cowen Park.
5.   Take the main path curving northeast into the Ravenna Park Trail. Follow the trail through the park.
6.   At the park's southeast end, turn east on NE 55th St.
7.   Turn south on 30th Ave. NE, which merges into Union Bay Pl. NE, to NE 45th St.
8.   Take a #65 bus from here to the University District; or cross the University Village mall to 25th Ave. NE and NE 47th St. and take a #68 bus (Monday through Saturday only) back to NE 65th St.

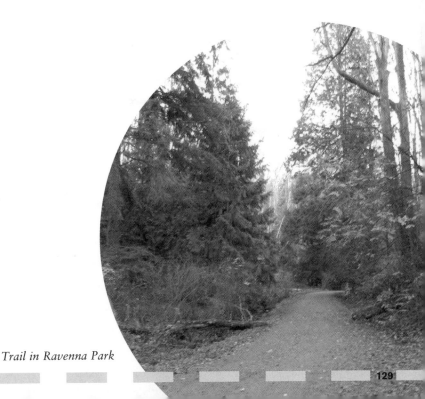

Trail in Ravenna Park

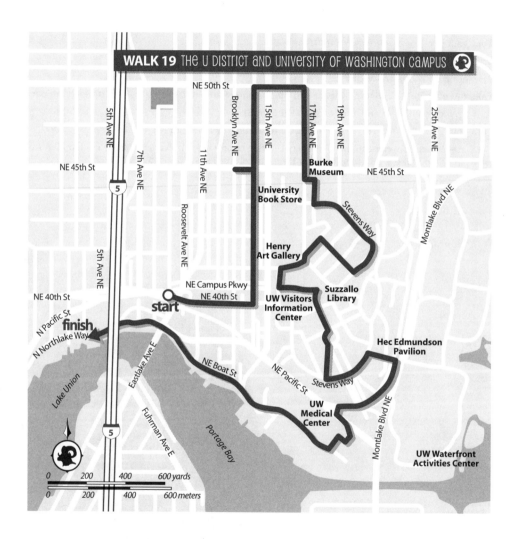

NE 50th St

5th Ave NE

Brooklyn Ave NE

15th Ave NE

17th Ave NE

19th Ave NE

25th Ave NE

NE 45th St

7th Ave NE

11th Ave NE

Roosevelt Ave NE

Burke
Museum

NE 45th St

Montlake Blvd NE

University
Book Store

Stevens Way

Henry
Art Gallery

5th Ave NE

NE Campus Pkwy
NE 40th St

Suzzallo
Library

NE 40th St

start

UW Visitors
Information
Center

N Pacific St

finish

N Northlake Way

Eastlake Ave E

NE Boat St

NE Pacific St

Stevens Way

Hec Edmundson
Pavilion

Lake Union

Fuhrman Ave E

Portage Bay

UW
Medical
Center

Montlake Blvd NE

UW Waterfront
Activities Center

0   200   400   600 yards

0   200   400   600 meters

19 THE U DISTRICT AND UNIVERSITY OF WASHINGTON CAMPUS: MAKING THE GRADE

BOUNDARIES: NE 50th St., Montlake Blvd. NE, NE Boat St., and 5th Ave. NE
DISTANCE: 4¼ miles, in two segments
DIFFICULTY: Moderate (a slight incline at the start)
PARKING: Free street parking west of Roosevelt Way NE, metered street parking on and east of Roosevelt
PUBLIC TRANSIT: Metro routes #30, 31, 70, 71, 72, 73, and 74 stop near this walk's start.

The University of Washington is the biggest single college campus west of the Rockies—and one of the handsomest in the United States. It's a place of stunning structures amid land-scaped repose, designed around a sweeping view of Mt. Rainier. From Greek Row to the Quad to the Health Sciences Center, its major buildings comprise a thorough retrospective of late-19th- and 20th-century institutional architecture. Adjacent to the campus, and somewhat grungier looking, is the first Seattle neighborhood for thousands who arrived as students and remained in town. Its main retail strip is also the main off-campus retail strip, where you can spot students from around the world and hipster youths from around the metro area.

● Start at the north side of NE 40th St. and 9th Ave. NE, at the University Friends Meeting, a Quaker church with a clean minimalist look. One of its longtime members, naturalist and political activist Floyd Schmoe, led a drive in the 1990s to remake the vacant lot across 40th into Seattle Peace Park. Its centerpiece is a statue of Sadako Sasaki, a 12-year-old victim of the Hiroshima blast. She's depicted holding a paper crane, as part of a healing ritual.

● Walk east on 40th, under the University Bridge and past the massive Terry-Lander dormitories. At 40th and Brooklyn Ave. NE, the gently angular UW Ethnic Cultural Center faces the older concrete box of the Ethnic Cultural Theater.

● Turn left onto University Way NE. Everyone calls it "The Ave." It starts with the Tudor-style College Inn building. Built in 1909, it's now a European-style hotel with a pub in the basement and shops on street level. At the southwest corner of 41st and The

Ave., the UW's new Jones Playhouse preserves the 1931 facade of the old Seattle Repertory Playhouse.

The Ave.'s retail and restaurant row really starts north of 41st, with the Big Time brewpub and Shultzy's Sausage. Above 42nd, Bulldog News has periodicals from the world over, on real paper. At 43rd, the bistro Flowers recycles the cursive neon from a florist shop. The next block up, the Varsity Cinema's flashy marquee faces the University Book Store, the District's retail anchor. Besides books, it's got computers, art supplies, clothes, Husky logo trinkets, and CDs. The latter makes it one of the last of the District's once-numerous record shops.

● Turn west onto the south side of NE 45th St., toward another classic movie house, the Neptune. Across Brooklyn Ave. NE, the UW has taken over Safeco Insurance's former 22-story office tower. Across 45th from there is a snazzier high-rise, the art deco Deca (née Edmond Meany) Hotel, where every room is a corner room.

● Return to University Way and resume heading north. At the northeast corner of 45th and The Ave., classical terra-cotta covers the 1913 Wells Fargo (formerly University State) Bank building. The storefronts north of that are dominated by young-adult apparel and eats (the latter including Pagliacci Pizza and the Greek-style Continental Pastry Shop). There's also a pulsating street life, involving student-age folk in most every fashion style of the past three decades.

● Take a right onto the south side of NE 50th St. A short flight of steps leads to the Grand Illusion, a 49-seat movie theater on the second floor of a tiny retail building. In the 1970s, Seattle's reputation as an art-film-going town began here. If you'd like to stop now, you can catch a southbound bus at the southwest corner of 50th and The Ave.

● Still with us? Then continue east on 50th, past some big churches—University Christian, University Lutheran, Hillel House, and the evangelical City Church. The latter is in a brick former Christian Science church at 17th Ave. NE and 50th.

● Turn south on 17th, better known as Greek Row. It's a wide boulevard with a grassy median strip and big trees shading the fraternities and sororities. Cross 45th and enter the UW campus, where 17th becomes Memorial Way.

● To your right, the first campus building you see is the Burke Museum of Natural History and Culture. This trove of regional artifacts is the state's oldest museum, founded in 1885; the current building dates to 1962. Cross Memorial to the back of the Jacobsen Observatory, whose original 1895 telescope still watches the skies. Across a parking lot from the observatory's front side, the Hughes Penthouse Theatre is the oldest theatre-in-the-round auditorium in the United States.

● Walk south from the observatory. Take the first left turn, onto Stevens Way. It curves southeast, past Hutchinson Hall, one of the campus's Gothic palaces. Built in the '20s for women's athletics, it now houses the Drama Department. Farther down are Lewis and Clark halls, 1900-era brick fortresses built as the university's first dorms.

● Take a right turn at Clark Hall, onto Skagit Lane. To your right is the Music Building, part of the Liberal Arts Quadrangle. You might hear singers and pianists practicing in its studios. To your left is the Communications Building, where mass media is still taught as a paying profession. Next to it is Thomson Hall, with a bust in front honoring Sen. Henry "Scoop" Jackson, who funneled much federal research money to the UW. Its School of International Studies, based at Thomson, is now named for Jackson. Beyond that is the Grieg Garden, a former parking lot reclaimed as green space, surrounding a statue of the Norwegian composer.

● Turn right at Thomson Hall onto King Lane, walking northwest through the Quad, a rectangular lawn surrounded by seven spectacular Gothic buildings. It's especially striking during cherry blossom season. Continue past the Quad toward Denny Hall. The campus's oldest building (1895) looks like a limestone French chateau.

Totem poles in front of the Burke Museum

- Take a left at Denny Hall toward the red Romanesque Parrington Hall. Continue southwest from Parrington on George Washington Lane, which curves south at the Henry Art Gallery, a top contemporary exhibition center. Across the lane, the UW's visitors center is on the lower level of Odegaard Undergraduate Library (a '60s brutalist box known on campus as "UGL-Y").

- Turn east past a George Washington statue, up some wide stairs, and across the brick-paved Red Square (nobody calls it by its official name, "Central Plaza") to Suzzallo Library, the grandest yet most inviting of the UW's Gothic marvels. If the library's open, go in and see its magnificent lobby and grand staircase, leading to the spectacular Graduate Reading Room.

- From Suzzallo's south side (with Gerberding Hall's churchlike bell tower to your right), head southeast to Drumheller Fountain, also known as Frosh Pond. The shallow pool was the center point of the Alaska-Yukon-Pacific Exposition, a fair staged in 1909 to celebrate Seattle's "arrival" as a trade center. Walk around to Garfield Lane, in front of the Chemistry Building on the pond's southwest side.

- Take Garfield southwest to the Medicinal Herb Garden, a secluded green space with dozens of plant samples to observe but not touch.

- Turn left (east) on Stevens Way, across the Rainier Vista promenade, named for the mountain you'll see if it's nice out. Just east of that is the Sylvan Theater, a secluded green space with four Doric columns from the UW's original downtown building.

- Turn east on Snohomish Way, onto the Burke-Gilman Trail. From here you can look across a skybridge toward Husky basketball's home, Hec Edmundson Pavilion. (Nobody calls it by its new official name, "Bank of America Arena.")

- Turn right onto the Burke-Gilman, curving southwest. Try not to get run over by jogging ROTC squads while you look east toward Husky Stadium, home of the once-mighty UW football program. Just past the Triangle Parking Garage, take a side path down to NE Pacific St.; cross Pacific and walk southeast to the UW Medical Center's main entrance.

- Enter the Medical Center. Take a right turn at the lobby, through the main corridor with its impressive public art collection, toward a big sign reading PACIFIC ELEVATORS.

Descend to Level 1. Follow the signs to the Plaza Cafe; cut through the dining area and out the building's south side.

- Head northeast on Columbia Road, which becomes NE Boat St., hugging the Montlake Cut's north shore. You might glimpse a rowing practice, or a UW Oceanography lab boat.

- At the end of Boat St. turn west back onto Pacific, which becomes NE Northlake Way. Continue west on Northlake under the University Bridge and the I-5 Ship Canal Bridge. On Northlake's north side are two acclaimed eateries, Voula's Lakeshore Cafe and Northlake Pizza. On Northlake's south side at 5th Ave. NE are a small waterfront park and Ivar's Salmon House, designed to look like a Native longhouse.

- To return to your start, backtrack to Pacific and 7th Ave. NE. Go north on 7th; take the outdoor steps up to 40th St.

CONNECTING THE WALKS

This walk connects easily with four other walks. It ends three-quarters of a mile northeast of Walk 14's end and starts across the University Bridge from Walk 23's end. At 45th and University Way you're four blocks west of Walk 15. At 50th and University Way you're a half mile south of Walk 18.

POINTS OF INTEREST

Peace Park seattle.gov/parks, NE 40th St. and 9th Ave. NE

College Inn collegeinnseattle.com, 4000 University Way NE, 206-634-2307

University Book Store bookstore.washington.edu, 4326 University Way NE, 206-548-2500

Burke Museum of Natural History and Culture washington.edu/burkemuseum, NE 45th St. and 17th Ave. NE, 206-543-5590

Henry Art Gallery henryart.org, 15th Ave. NE and NE 41st St, 206-543-2280

University of Washington Visitors Center washington.edu/discover/visit, 4060 George Washington Lane, 206-543-9198

Suzzallo Library lib.washington.edu/suzzallo, UW Central Plaza, 206-543-0242

Hec Edmundson Pavilion gohuskies.com, 3870 Montlake Blvd. NE, 206-543-2200

UW Medical Center uwmedicine.washington.edu 1959 NE Pacific St., 206-598-3300

Ivar's Salmon House ivars.com, 401 NE Northlake Way, 206-632-0767

route summary

1. Start at the north side of NE 40th St. and 9th Ave. NE. Walk east on 40th.
2. Walk north on University Way NE.
3. Take a one-block detour west on NE 45th St. to Brooklyn Ave. NE.
4. Return to University Way, walking north.
5. Turn east on NE 50th St.
6. Turn south on 17th Ave. NE into the UW campus.
7. Turn east toward the Hughes Penthouse Theatre. Walk south along a parking lot.
8. Turn east on Stevens Way, then curving southeast.
9. Turn southwest on Skagit Lane.
10. Turn northwest on King Lane through the Quad.
11. Turn southwest on Klickitat Lane, which doglegs into George Washington Lane and curves south.
12. Turn east through Red Square.
13. Walk east past Suzzallo Library's south side.
14. Walk around Drumheller Fountain to Garfield Lane.
15. Turn southwest on Garfield Lane.
16. Turn east on Stevens Way, curving north.
17. Turn southeast on Snohomish Way.
18. Turn southwest on the Burke-Gilman Trail.
19. Take a side path down to NE Pacific St. Cross Pacific and walk southeast to the UW Medical Center.
20. Enter the Medical Center. Turn right at the lobby, to a bank of elevators. Descend to Level 1. Follow the signs to the Plaza Cafe. Exit through the cafe's south side.
21. Head northeast on Columbia Road, which doglegs into NE Boat St.
22. Turn west onto Pacific, which becomes NE Northlake Way, to 5th Ave. NE.

Suzzallo Library

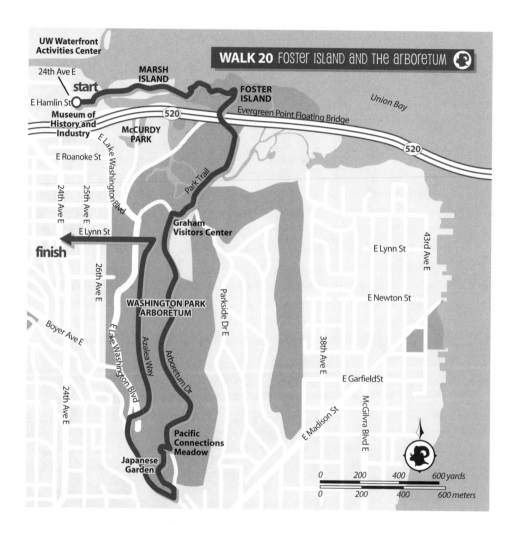

UW Waterfront
Activities Center

24th Ave E

start

E Hamlin St

Museum of
History and
Industry

**MARSH
ISLAND**

**FOSTER
ISLAND**

Evergreen Point Floating Bridge

Union Bay

WALK 20 FOSTER ISLAND AND THE ARBORETUM

520

**McCURDY
PARK**

E Lake Washington Blvd

E Roanoke St

24th Ave E

25th Ave E

E Lynn St

Park Trail

**Graham
Visitors Center**

520

E Lynn St

43rd Ave E

finish

26th Ave E

E Newton St

**WASHINGTON PARK
ARBORETUM**

Parkside Dr E

E Lake Washington Blvd

Boyer Ave E

Azalea Way

Arboretum Dr

38th Ave E

E Garfield St

24th Ave E

McGilvra Blvd E

E Madison St

**Pacific
Connections
Meadow**

**Japanese
Garden**

0   200   400   600 yards

0   200   400   600 meters

20 FOSTER ISLAND AND THE ARBORETUM: THE TREE MUSEUM

BOUNDARIES: 24th Ave. E., E. Hamlin St., Arboretum Dr. E., and Lake Washington Blvd. E.
DISTANCE: 3½ miles
DIFFICULTY: Easy (one gentle incline)
PARKING: Free parking at the MOHAI lot (except on UW football game days)
PUBLIC TRANSIT: Metro routes #43 and 48 stop near this walk's start.

Washington Park Arboretum, jointly run by the City of Seattle and UW, is a 230-acre plant museum disguised as a nature corridor and a popular get-away-from-it-all spot. You don't need to be a scholar of plant science to enjoy it; you simply need a pair of feet and an attentive eye. This route takes you into the arboretum via a unique walk along the water, through a pair of artificial islets. At the heart of your walk are two beautifully meditative areas, an elaborate Japanese garden and an open meadow honoring the Pacific Rim's diverse flora.

● Start at the Museum of History and Industry in McCurdy Park, 24th Ave. E. and E. Hamlin St. Sometimes called "Seattle's attic," it's a highly accessible source to the city's short but colorful heritage. (Note: MOHAI plans to move from here to Lake Union Park, Walk 6, sometime in 2012.)

● Walk east through MOHAI's east parking lot, to the Marsh Island footbridge. Much of the following path is on a boardwalk, or "floating trail." It winds east through, well, marshes, with plenty of nesting birds (wrens and blackbirds in summer, crows in winter). This little piece of nature was made by people, like so much in this city of nature. It was transformed from shallow waters to a flat islet early last century, when Lake Washington and Lake Union were lowered several feet.

● Take the trail across another wooden bridge and onto larger Foster Island. This bridge, and the subsequent stretch of boardwalk along Foster's north side, offer great water-level views of Union Bay. You can see pleasure boats, canoes, rowing crews, and waterfowl; in the distance are Husky Stadium and the upscale Laurelhurst neighborhood. The boardwalk becomes a dirt trail, which leads to a crossroads. Turn right.

- Follow this path south under the 520 freeway and into the arboretum proper. This area of bending creeks and tiny islets is popular with canoeists; you can become one temporarily by renting from the UW's Waterfront Activities Center, located near the stadium.

- One short footbridge later, you're off Foster Island and back on the mainland. The trail soon leads to a paved street, Broadmoor Dr. E. To your left you can peer in at the private Broadmoor Golf and Country Club. Beyond that you might see some mansion roofs from the gated Broadmoor residential community.

- Turn left onto Arboretum Dr. E. To your left you soon see the Graham Visitors Center, where you can get a detailed map of the arboretum and all its plant and tree samples. A greenhouse complex is just south of that. From this point, the road becomes pedestrian only, winding gently uphill. Despite its "natural" appearance, this area was completely logged in the late 19th century by the Puget Mill Co. The City of Seattle acquired the land in 1900. In 1934, the city brought in UW as its partner in developing the arboretum, with the help of Works Progress Administration (WPA) laborers.

  Continue strolling along Arboretum Dr. You catch occasional glimpses of the golf course behind the fence to your left. In closer view, you see displays of Japanese and Asiatic maples, magnolias, mountain ashes, birches, poplars, legumes, camellias, rhododendrons, and witch hazel plants. More than 12,000 plants are in the arboretum's official collection.

- Eventually you reach a clearing to your right, the Pacific Connections Meadow, the arboretum's newest attraction that features a circular gravel path. Take a right turn onto the circle, going counterclockwise. Surrounding it are gardens representing different Pacific Rim places—Australia, New Zealand, China, Chile, and Cascadia (the United States and Canadian Northwest).

- Just before the circle returns to Arboretum Dr., take a right onto the Cascadia Forest Trail. It wends a very indirect path through locally native trees and plants and leads to stone-paved steps, switchbacking downhill.

- At the bottom of this trail, take a right turn back onto Arboretum Dr. To your left you find a stone cottage. Built by the WPA, it serves as both a symbolic gatehouse and as a residence for the park's security chief. From here, you can continue on Arboretum Dr. out of the park and onto the Madison Valley retail strip.

- If you're continuing with us, take a sharp right turn onto Lake Washington Blvd. E. On your left, you soon see the Seattle Japanese Garden. Since 1960, this exquisite formal garden has entranced and relaxed thousands with its artfully placed ponds, paths, bridges, lanterns, shrubs, and flowers. The garden has a $5 adult admission fee ($3 for kids, seniors, and the disabled). It's closed in winter.

- North of the Japanese Garden on Lake Washington Blvd., take a right turn onto a short parking strip that leads to Azalea Way. Wind north on Azalea. In some stretches, it's a gravel path. In others, it's a wide grassy promenade. Those parts can be muddy during and after long rains. Along both sides are many more tree and plant samples, identified with handy signs. The tree samples alone include the holly, ash, walnut, hawthorne, and (yes, Monty Python viewers) the larch.

- Azalea eventually leads to a crossroads, where you can see the visitors center to your right. Take a left instead. Cross the Wilcox Footbridge, a narrow concrete-and-brick archway over Lake Washington Blvd. It looks fancier than a pedestrian overpass needs to be for a reason. An aboveground sewer pipe is hidden inside all that stone-work. Continue west and out of the arboretum.

- Continue west on E. Lynn St. back to 24th. There's a little retail strip with a coffee-house, a convenience store, a couple of moderately priced restaurants, and a damn cute antique and curio shop. You can walk up 24th back to your start, or take a #43 or 48 bus.

CONNECTING THE WALKS

This walk connects easily with three other walks. It starts three-quarters of a mile south of Walk 19, across the Montlake Bridge. It ends a quarter mile north of Walk 23. At Arboretum Dr. and Lake Washington Blvd. you're a half mile southwest of Walk 21.

POINTS OF INTEREST

Museum of History and Industry seattlehistory.org, 2700 24th Ave. E., 206-234-1126

UW Waterfront Activities Center depts.washington.edu/ima/IMA_wac.php, 3900 Montlake Blvd. NE, 206-534-9433

Washington Park Arboretum depts.washington.edu/uwbg/gardens/wpa.shtml, 2300 Arboretum Dr. E., 206-543-8800

Seattle Japanese Garden seattle.gov/parks, 1075 Lake Washington Blvd. E., 206-684-4725

ROUTE SUMMARY

1. Start at the Museum of History and Industry in McCurdy Park, 24th Ave. E. and E. Hamlin St.
2. Walk east through MOHAI's east parking lot, to the Marsh Island footbridge.
3. Cross onto Marsh Island. Take the trail east across Marsh to another bridge and onto Foster Island.
4. Continue on the park trail, turning south at the crossroads.
5. Follow the path under the 520 freeway, then across a short footbridge onto the mainland.
6. Turn left onto Arboretum Dr. E. Wind south past the Graham Visitors Center, to Pacific Connections Meadow.
7. Take the Cascadia Forest Trail from Pacific Connections Meadow's south side, switchbacking downhill back to Arboretum Dr.
8. Turn right onto Arboretum Dr.
9. Turn right onto Lake Washington Blvd. E.
10. North of the Seattle Japanese Garden, take a right onto a parking strip that leads to Azalea Way.
11. Wind north on Azalea back toward the visitors center.
12. Turn west, across the Wilcox Footbridge and out of the arboretum.
13. Continue west on E. Lynn St. back to 24th.

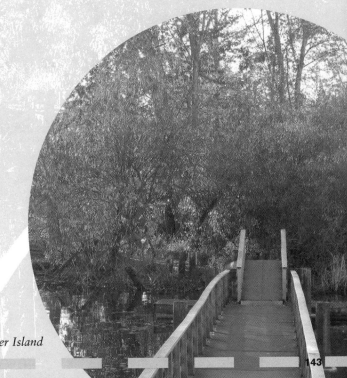

Wooden bridge to Foster Island

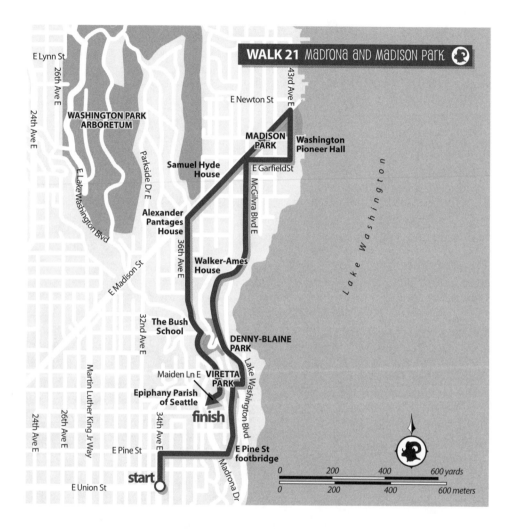

E Lynn St

26th Ave E

24th Ave E

WASHINGTON PARK ARBORETUM

Parkside Dr E

E Lake Washington Blvd

E Madison St

32nd Ave E

36th Ave E

Martin Luther King Jr Way

24th Ave E

26th Ave E

34th Ave E

E Newton St

43rd Ave E

MADISON PARK

Washington Pioneer Hall

Samuel Hyde House

E Garfield St

McGilvra Blvd E

Alexander Pantages House

Walker-Ames House

Lake Washington

The Bush School

DENNY-BLAINE PARK

Maiden Ln E   **VIRETTA PARK**

Lake Washington Blvd

Epiphany Parish of Seattle

finish

E Pine St

start

E Union St

E Pine St footbridge

Madrona Dr

0   200   400   600 yards

0   200   400   600 meters

21 Madrona and Madison Park: Gracious Living by a Lake

BOUNDARIES: **34th Ave., E. Union St., 43rd Ave. E., and E. Madison St.**
DISTANCE: **3¾ miles, in two segments**
DIFFICULTY: **Moderate (one rather long uphill stretch)**
PARKING: **Free parking on 34th Ave. E. and adjoining streets**
PUBLIC TRANSIT: **Metro routes #2 and 3 stop near this walk's start.**

Seattle's eastern slopes overlooking Lake Washington contain some of the city's grandest residences. This portion of the lakefront and vicinity also offers big and small parks, a pioneers' meeting hall, gay and lesbian sunbathers, and Seattle's only (unofficial) Kurt Cobain memorial. Your walk starts amid some popular bistros, then follows a narrow wooden bridge over a ravine. At its middle is Madison Park, a former enclave of summer cottages that's now a self-contained town within the city.

● Start at 34th Ave. and E. Union St., center of the Madrona business district. It's got a handful of quaint, comfy eateries. One favorite is the Hi-Spot Cafe, a breakfast and lunch place in a 1904 Victorian home. Weekend brunch lines here often stretch onto the sidewalk. Walk north on 34th two blocks to E. Pine St.

● Turn east on Pine to 37th Ave., past some classic upper-middle-class housing stock. Continue as Pine becomes a pedestrian-only path for three blocks, alternating between sidewalks and downhill stairs between some dense trees, to Madrona Dr.

● On the east side of Madrona Dr., Pine turns into a wooden pedestrian bridge over a deep, lush ravine. It's reminiscent of the trestles that once bore trolley cars rattling down to Lake Washington. This bridge has a turnoff in the middle, a secondary bridge leading left. But keep going straight, to Pine and Evergreen Pl. There's a light pole right in the middle of your way at the bridge's east end, which helps discourage motorcyclists from crossing it.

- Wind north on Evergreen, barely wider than an alley. In two blocks it widens (slightly) into 39th Ave. E. It's surrounded by dense trees and shrubbery, hiding the homes of the affluent and reclusive. One of these, to your right, is the former home of Starbucks boss Howard Schultz. You can tell it by the private driveway Schultz had added, cutting through the city-owned Viretta Park.

- Enter Viretta, descend some stairs, and walk east through the small neighborhood park. Near its center is an ordinary wood-and-metal bench covered in etched graffiti and often adorned with flowers. This is "Kurt's Bench," still a gathering place for fans of singer-songwriter Kurt Cobain. On the day in 1994 when Cobain's death was announced, this spot was the closest the public could get to the garage (since demolished) where he'd died. These fans have unofficially nicknamed Viretta "Kurt's Park."

- From Viretta Park's eastern end, head north along Lake Washington Blvd. To your right you see the entrance to another small park, Denny-Blaine. It's a grassy strip that leads to a short public beach. In the 1990s, lesbians from Capitol Hill would defiantly sunbathe topless here. That's less common now, but local GLBTs still frequent the beach.

- Just north of Denny-Blaine is a five-way intersection. Take a soft right onto McGilvra Blvd. E., winding north. The lakefront along this stretch is all private. You can see massive view homes to your left, and old mansions and newer McMansions (or peekaboo pieces of them, or just their garages) to your right.

- McGilvra curves northeast, then north again as it passes the quite exclusive Seattle Tennis Club. It's said to have a decade-long waiting list for membership. North of there, McGilvra traverses inland, blocks without views and with significantly smaller houses. Some of these lots were originally platted as summer homes for the affluent.

- Turn east at E. Garfield St. for three blocks. On the south side of Garfield and 42nd Ave. E., a fence encloses but doesn't conceal a little private residential enclave. It was originally the estate of Judge John McGilvra, one of the neighborhood's initial developers. During the Great Depression, its then-owners turned it into a small gated community, with several smaller homes in place of McGilvra's mansion.

- Turn north on 43rd Ave. E. To your right, three residential towers stand on the site of an old amusement pier Judge McGilvra had built to stimulate land sales in the neighborhood. North of those is the brick facade of Washington Pioneer Hall, home for a century to the Pioneer Association of the State of Washington. North of that lies Madison Park itself, a stretch of lakefront donated by McGilvra to the city as a public amenity for residents of his developments.

- Take a hard left onto E. Madison St., heading southwest through the Madison Park business strip. It's a pleasant stroll past sidewalk cafes, fashionable boutiques, and even a few practical places like a small supermarket and a hardware store. One of the oldest spots here is the Red Onion Tavern, a cozy bar with crimson wallpaper, a fireplace, and hearty pizzas.

- Continue southwest on Madison beyond the business district, heading uphill past some very fancy homes. The fanciest is the Samuel Hyde House, a brick edifice with a white Corinthian portico. It's now the Russian consul general's residence. Beyond it stand the wrought-iron fences surrounding Broadmoor, the city's oldest and poshest gated development. Near 36th Ave. E. you see a fancy brick bus shelter outside the fence, built by Broadmoor for its residents' household staffs.

- Turn south on 36th, continuing uphill. To your immediate right is the Alexander Pantages House. Built in 1909 by a vaudeville-theater mogul, it has two stories of white plaster beneath a red-tile roof. Three blocks later, at the northeast corner of 36th and E. Valley St., is the big brick Walker-Ames House, official residence of the UW president. After crossing E. Mercer St., 36th transforms from a wide landscaped boulevard into a one-lane side street, winding downhill toward Lake Washington Blvd. E.

- Turn southeast on Lake Washington Blvd. and continue for one block. To your left you see a 1917 Tudor mansion behind a short uphill driveway. It's part of the Bush School, a K–12 private academy.

- Take a right onto 37th Ave. E., which curves southeast and becomes Dorffel Dr. E., another narrow tree-lined street. You see other historic houses, and brief glimpses of the lake views these houses were built to exploit. When it forks with E. John St., keep right to stay on Dorffel.

● Then take the next right fork, going southwest onto Maiden Ln. E. for one block, back to Madrona Dr. Turn right on Madrona. To your left you see the sprawling Epiphany Parish. The Episcopal church's chapel (its easternmost building) was designed in 1911 by noted local architect Ellsworth Storey. To your right you see another spectacular brick bus shelter, a remnant from the prewar trolley days. Here you can catch a #2 bus back to 34th and Union.

CONNECTING THE WALKS

This walk connects easily to two other walks. At 36th and Madison you're a half mile northeast of Walk 20. At Pine and Madrona Dr. you're 1 mile north of Walk 29.

POINTS OF INTEREST

Hi-Spot Cafe hispotcafe.com, 1410 34th Ave., 206-325-7905

Viretta Park seattle.gov/parks, 39th Ave. E. and E. John St.

Denny-Blaine Park seattle.gov/parks, 200 Lake Washington Blvd. E.

Madison Park seattle.gov/parks, E. Madison St. and E. Howe St.

Washington Pioneer Hall wapioneers.org, 1642 43rd Ave.

Red Onion Tavern 4210 E. Madison St., 206-323-1611

Samuel Hyde House 3726 E. Madison St.

Alexander Pantages House 1117 36th Ave. E.

Bush School bush.edu, 405 36th Ave. E., 206-322-7978

Epiphany Parish of Seattle epiphanyseattle.org, 1805 38th Ave., 206-324-2573

route summary

1. Start on 34th Ave., walking north from E. Union St.

2. Turn east on E. Pine St. to 37th Ave.

3. Continue on Pine as it becomes a pedestrian-only path.

4. Cross the footbridge from Madrona Dr. to E. Pine St. and Evergreen Pl.

5. Wind north on Evergreen Pl., which becomes 39th Ave. E.

6. Cut east through Viretta Park to Lake Washington Blvd. E.

7. Wind north along Lake Washington Blvd.

8. Take a soft right onto McGilvra Blvd. E., winding northeast then north.

9. Turn east onto E. Garfield St.

10. Turn north on 43rd Ave. E.

11. Turn southwest on E. Madison St.

12. Turn south on 36th Ave. E.

13. Turn southeast on Lake Washington Blvd.

14. Take a right onto 37th Ave. E., which turns into Dorffel Dr. E., winding southeast.

15. Turn southwest on Maiden Ln. E., back to Madrona Dr.

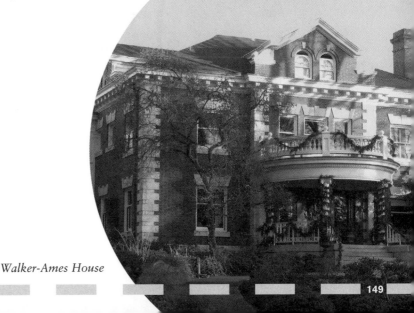

Walker-Ames House

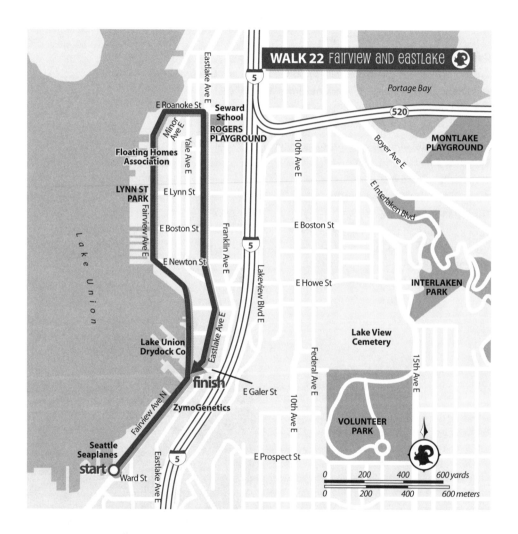

WALK 22 Fairview and Eastlake

Portage Bay

520

MONTLAKE
PLAYGROUND

E Roanoke St

Eastlake Ave E

Seward
School
ROGERS
PLAYGROUND

Minor Ave E

Yale Ave E

Floating Homes
Association

LYNN ST
PARK

E Lynn St

Fairview Ave E

E Boston St

E Newton St

Franklin Ave E

10th Ave E

E Boston St

E Howe St

Boyer Ave E

E Interlaken Blvd

INTERLAKEN
PARK

L a k e   U n i o n

Lakeview Blvd E

Lake View
Cemetery

Lake Union
Drydock Co

Eastlake Ave E

finish

E Galer St

Federal Ave E

10th Ave E

15th Ave E

Fairview Ave N

ZymoGenetics

VOLUNTEER
PARK

Seattle
Seaplanes

start

Eastlake Ave E

5

Ward St

E Prospect St

0   200   400   600 yards

0   200   400   600 meters

22 Fairview and Eastlake: Gracious Living on a Lake

BOUNDARIES: **Fairview Ave. E., Ward St., Eastlake Ave. E., and E. Roanoke St.**
DISTANCE: **2¼ miles**
DIFFICULTY: **Easy (one short uphill stretch)**
PARKING: **Pay lot at Fairview and Yale Ave. N.**
PUBLIC TRANSIT: **Metro route #70 and the Lake Union Streetcar stop near this walk's start.**

In old Japan, the term "floating world" referred to nomadic aristocrats, untethered to the land or to the rural economy. In Seattle, it's a close-knit subculture of a few hundred affluent households in houseboats, as glorified in the film *Sleepless in Seattle*. About half of these houseboats are moored along Lake Union's east side, indirectly but securely attached to the urban shore. This walk gets you as close to these dockside abodes as you can legally get. You'll also see kayaks, seaplanes, a restored former power plant, and the city's oldest public school.

● Start on the west side of Fairview Ave. N. at Ward St., walking northeast along Lake Union. To your left, the northern reaches of the South Lake Union restaurant strip are mixed in with yacht moorage docks. You soon find a few steps to descend, onto a floating sidewalk over an inlet. To your right is the former Lake Union Steam Plant, built by Seattle City Light between 1912 and 1928. It's now headquarters for the biotech company ZymoGenetics. As part of the remodel, the plant's tall smokestacks were replaced by lightweight replicas.

● Once you're back on solid ground, the Seattle Seaplanes dock appears to your left. If you've got the money, they'll take you on a 20-minute scenic flight. Fairview forks here with Eastlake Ave. E. Keep left to stay on Fairview.

The next long pier complex up ahead is home to the Lake Union Drydock Co. The shipyard and boat-repair facility is one of the last remnants of Lake Union's heritage as a "working lake." Another is the National Oceanic and Atmospheric Administration's Marine Operations Center, which used the next pier north as a winter home for its research ships—until a 2006 fire rendered the dock unusable. They're now moored elsewhere around town. NOAA now wants to move the whole regional operation, including a land-based laboratory, to Oregon.

North of that, the houseboat docks start. These aren't boats; they're houses on rafts, semipermanently moored to their docks. Seattle has about 500 floating-home moorage slots, down from more than 2,000 in the 1940s. Increased demand and limited supply have mostly turned them from artsy bohemian digs into the upscale professional abodes seen in the film *Sleepless in Seattle*.

On the east side of Fairview at E. Lynn St. you can get refreshments at Pete's Wines, formerly Pete's Supermarket. As the nomenclature implies, it's evolved over the past four decades from a grocery with a good wine selection to a major wine shop with a fair grocery selection. You can consume nonalcoholic purchases across the street at Lynn Street Park, a lakefront mini-park first established by the store's founder Pete Omalanz. It's festooned with tile art pieces, the product of a 2003 community campaign. Some of the tiles depict the joys of wine in memory of the late *Seattle Times* wine critic and houseboat resident Tom Stockley. Neighbors fought the Seattle Parks Department to keep those tiles installed.

A short bit north of the park, the Floating Homes Association (a houseboat owners' advocacy group) operates a volunteer-run gift shop, the Houseboatique. Here you can buy posters and books about houseboats, and learn about the lifestyle and its hundred-year history.

● This stretch of Fairview ends with a right turn onto E. Roanoke St. To your left, you see some more houseboat docks, plus some ritzy new lakefront townhomes. Three moderately uphill blocks later, you're at Eastlake Ave. E., the neighborhood's main arterial. Across from you is Rogers Playground. Behind that is Seward School, the Seattle School District's oldest extant site. It now houses an alternative elementary program, The Options Program at Seward (TOPS).

● Turn south on Eastlake. This street, once little more than a byway between downtown and the U District, saw a lot of redevelopment during the 2000s. It's now dotted with recent office, apartment, and mixed-use structures. Among the surviving older businesses here are the 14 Carrot Cafe (a hippie-esque bistro), the Eastlake Zoo Tavern (a hippie-esque bar, more spacious and more brightly lit than most), and Patrick's Fly Shop (fishing gear). Tiles embedded in Eastlake's sidewalks depict indigenous local plants and insects.

South of Eastlake and E. Howe St. is the Bonneville Broadcasting Building, home to longtime news-talk leader KIRO-FM. A short detour east on Howe leads to a long set of outdoor steps, heading under the Interstate 5 overpass and up the west slope of Capitol Hill (Walk 25).

● Take a right at Eastlake and E. Galer St., returning to Fairview just north of the old steam plant. Backtrack south on Fairview to your start, or take a #70 bus.

CONNECTING THE WALKS

The walk connects easily to two other walks. It starts at Walk 6's midpoint. Its midpoint is a half mile south of Walk 23's end.

POINTS OF INTEREST

ZymoGenetics zymogenetics.com, 1201 Eastlake Ave. E.

Seattle Seaplanes seattleseaplanes.com, 1325 Fairview Ave. E., 206-329-9638

Lake Union Drydock Co. ludd.com, 1515 Fairview Ave. E.

Lynn Street Park seattle.gov/parks, Fairview Ave. E. and E. Lynn St.

Pete's Wines peteswineshop.com, 58 E. Lynn St., 206-322-2660

Floating Homes Association seattlefloatinghomes.org, 2329 Fairview Ave. E., 206-325-1132

Seward School and Rogers Playground topsk8.org, 2500 Franklin Ave. E.

14 Carrot Cafe 2305 Eastlake Ave. E., 206-324-1442

Eastlake Zoo Tavern eastlakezoo.com, 2301 Eastlake Ave. E., 206-329-3277

Patrick's Fly Shop patricksflyshop.com, 2237 Eastlake Ave. E., 206-325-8988

route summary

1. Start at Fairview Ave. N. and Ward St., walking northeast along Lake Union.
2. At the fork with Eastlake Ave. E., keep left to stay on Fairview.
3. At Fairview's northern end, turn east on E. Roanoke St.
4. Turn south on Eastlake.
5. Turn east on E. Galer St. to return to Fairview.

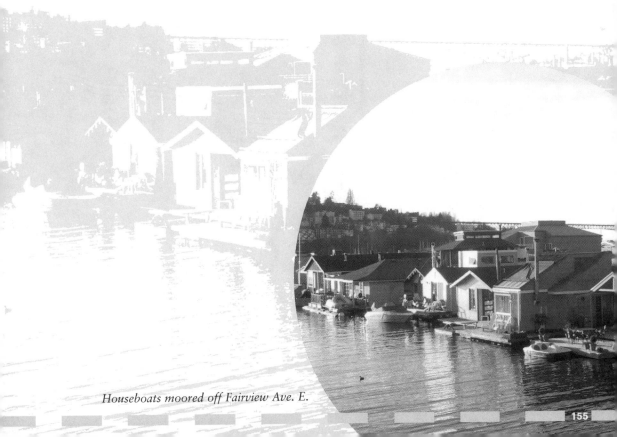

Houseboats moored off Fairview Ave. E.

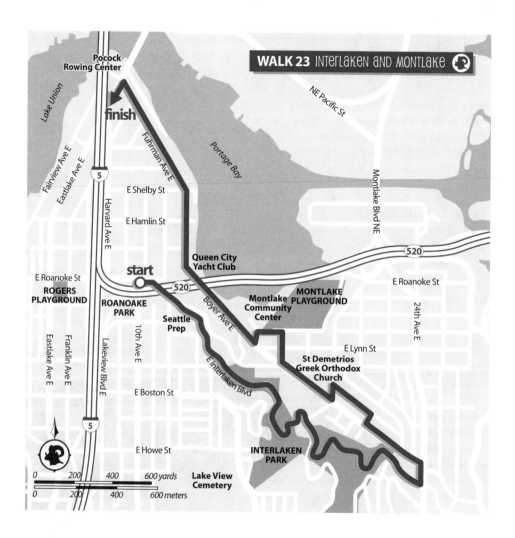

Pocock Rowing Center

Lake Union

finish

Fairview Ave E

Eastlake Ave E

Harvard Ave E

Fuhrman Ave E

E Shelby St

E Hamlin St

Portage Bay

NE Pacific St

Montlake Blvd NE

Queen City Yacht Club

start

E Roanoke St

ROGERS PLAYGROUND

ROANOAKE PARK

Lakeview Blvd E

10th Ave E

Seattle Prep

Boyer Ave E

Montlake Community Center

MONTLAKE PLAYGROUND

E Roanoke St

24th Ave E

Franklin Ave E

Eastlake Ave E

E Interlaken Blvd

E Lynn St

St Demetrios Greek Orthodox Church

E Boston St

E Howe St

INTERLAKEN PARK

Lake View Cemetery

0   200   400   600 yards
0   200   400   600 meters

23 INTerLaKeN aND MONTLaKe: aN UrBaN WiLDerNeSS

BOUNDARIES: 10th Ave. E., E. Interlaken Blvd., 24th Ave. E., Boyer Ave. E., and Eastlake Ave. E.
DISTANCE: 3½ miles
DIFFICULTY: Easy (mostly flat or downhill)
PARKING: Free street parking on 10th Ave. E. (north of E. Roanoke St.)
PUBLIC TRANSIT: Metro route #49 stops near this walk's start.

Interlaken Boulevard is one of the Olmsted plan's (Walk 24) promenades through the city. Before that, in the 1890s, it was part of a bicycle-path network that crossed Seattle in the pre-Model T years. It remains a great place to retreat from the big city and commune with the big trees. Like Ravenna Park (Walk 18), Interlaken lets you pretend you're out in a deep wilderness, without the wasteful fuel consumption of a real country road trip. Beneath this path, the Montlake neighborhood sports some modestly sized but stately homes, and one grand midcentury-modern church.

- Start at E. Roanoke St., going east from 10th Ave. E. Pass the south end of Roanoke Park, a nice little neighborhood green space.

- Turn southwest onto Delmar Dr. E. After you cross an overpass above State Highway 520, you get a peek to your right of Seattle Prep, a Jesuit high school with a '50s-modern look.

- Take a soft right onto E. Interlaken Blvd. You're immediately twisting your way through Interlaken Park. You're walking up, then down Capitol Hill's steep northeast slope. Tall trees on either side of this narrow, curving street block most views of anything beyond them. Some of these second-growth trees are up to a century old. There are even a few old-growth redwoods in the mix. It all makes for a spectacular interplay of light and shadow, especially on a sunny late afternoon. Cars are allowed on this part of the boulevard, but you won't see many of them. As the road U-turns north, you find a small plaque mounted on a rock to your right that honors Louisa Boren Denny, one of Seattle's founding white settlers.

- Shortly after that the boulevard forks with Interlaken Dr. E. Take a left to continue on E. Interlaken Blvd. After another U-turn south, there's an intersection with 19th Ave. E. Cars have to turn onto 19th, but you can keep going straight as the boulevard becomes restricted to pedestrians and bicycles. Along this half-mile stretch you can more clearly hear the birds and feel one with the flora and fauna. Reality intrudes at an intersection with 21st Ave. E., as cars rejoin you on the boulevard. Soon after that you're heading out of the park and back into civilization.

- Turn north onto 24th Ave. E; then immediately turn northwest onto Boyer Ave. E. To your right you soon spot Boyer Children's Clinic, providing both therapy and schooling to kids with neuromuscular disorders. The handsome 1991 brick structure includes some nice public art and signs done up in a grownup designer's idea of kids' handwriting.

- Two residential blocks later, dogleg right onto 22nd Ave. E., for the first of two digressions off of Boyer. Take an immediate left onto E. Blaine St. The homes here take on a storybook feel. Mostly built in the late 1920s, they range from English cottages to Tudor A-frames. Blaine ends at 19th Ave. E., with the grand dome and cupola of Saint Demetrios Greek Orthodox Church. Built in 1962, the modern-yet-traditional building was designed by Paul Thiry, one of the Seattle World's Fair's chief architects. Take a left-right dogleg around the church and back onto Boyer.

- Resume going northwest on Boyer to 16th Ave. E., where we make our second digression. Heading north on 16th, you see some more exquisite brick Tudor homes. Then 16th ends at E. Calhoun St., by the Montlake Playground and Community Center. The latter occupies two buildings. The older building is an extra-large version of the Tudor cottage architecture you've already seen in the neighborhood.

- Turn west on Calhoun, which quickly becomes a pedestrian-only path. Turn south on 15th Ave. E. for one block, back to Boyer. Resume going northwest on Boyer's north side, under Highway 520. Interspersed among the tasteful old homes here are some boxy new townhomes.

- As Boyer curves from northwest to north, the Queen City Yacht Club shows up on your right. The long, low clubhouse you see from the street extends for two more stories below. The members-only moorage slips can accommodate more than 200 boats. The club sponsors a parade of lighted boats around Seattle's waterways every Christmas season.

- Continue as Boyer bends northwest again, becoming Fuhrman Ave. E., bending northwest. You get glimpses of Portage Bay and the Montlake Cut between houses. Just before the intersection with Eastlake Ave. E. at the south end of the University Bridge are two classic UW student watering holes. To your right is the former Red Robin Tavern, which became the flagship of the national burger chain of the same name before it closed in 2010. To your left is a Tudor-style mini-castle. It's now part of the regional Romio's Pizza chain; its former identities include Scoundrel's Lair, Rapunzel's, and the Llahngaelhyn (a 1960s jazz club). Just beyond Eastlake is the Pocock Rowing Center, the region's top rowing club and school.

- Turn southwest onto the east side of Eastlake for one block, past the artisan bakery Le Fournil. Then take a soft left onto Harvard Ave. E. From here you can take a half-mile uphill trek back to Roanoke Avenue.

CONNECTING THE WALKS

The walk connects easily with three other walks. It starts five blocks east of Walk 22. Its midpoint is three blocks north of Walk 20's end. It ends across the University Bridge from Walk 19's start.

POINTS OF INTEREST

Roanoke Park seattle.gov/parks, 2409 10th Ave. E.

Seattle Preparatory School seaprep.org, 2400 11th Ave. E., 206-325-2400

Interlaken Park seattle.gov/parks, 2451 Delmar Ave. E.

St. Demetrios Greek Orthodox Church saintdemetrios.com, 2100 Boyer Ave. E., 206-325-4347

Montlake Playground and Community Center seattle.gov/parks, 1618 E. Calhoun St., 206-684-4736

Queen City Yacht Club queencity.org, 2608 Boyer Ave. E., 206-709-2000

Pocock Rowing Center pocockrowingcenter.org, 3320 Fuhrman Ave. E., 206-328-0778

Romio's Pizza romios-pizza.com, 3242 Eastlake Ave. E., 206-322-4453

route summary

1. Start at E. Roanoke St., walking east from 10th Ave. E.
2. Turn southwest on Delmar Dr. E.
3. Take a soft right on E. Interlaken Blvd., winding southeast through Interlaken Park.
4. At the fork with Interlaken Dr. E., take a left to continue on E. Interlaken Blvd., heading out of the park.
5. Turn north on 24th Ave. E.
6. Turn northwest on Boyer Ave. E.
7. Turn right on 22nd Ave. E.
8. Turn left on E. Blaine St.
9. Turn south on 19th Ave. E.
10. Resume going northwest on Boyer.
11. Dogleg north on 16th Ave. E.
12. Turn west on E. Calhoun St.
13. Turn south on 15th Ave. E.
14. Return to Boyer, bending north.
15. Continue as Boyer becomes Fuhrman Ave. E., bending northwest.
16. Turn southwest at Eastlake Ave. E., to Harvard Ave. E.

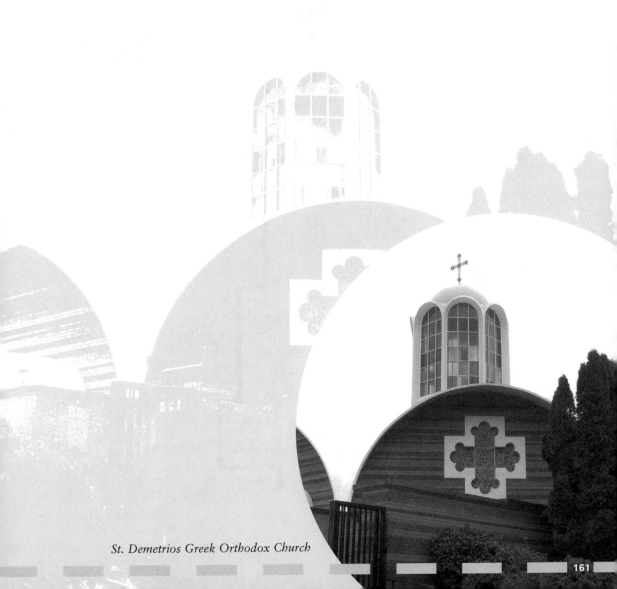

St. Demetrios Greek Orthodox Church

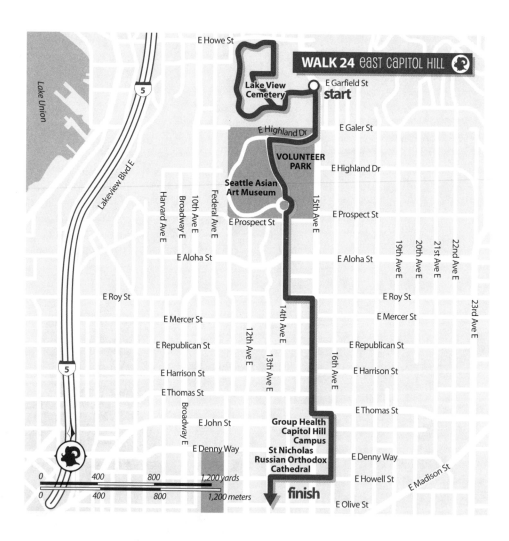

E Howe St

WALK 24 east capitol hill

Lake Union

5

E Garfield St
start

Lake View
Cemetery

Lakeview Blvd E

E Highland Dr

E Galer St

VOLUNTEER
PARK

E Highland Dr

Seattle Asian
Art Museum

Harvard Ave E

10th Ave E

Broadway E

Federal Ave E

E Prospect St

15th Ave E

E Prospect St

E Aloha St

E Aloha St

19th Ave E

20th Ave E

21st Ave E

22nd Ave E

E Roy St

E Roy St

23rd Ave E

5

E Mercer St

E Mercer St

E Republican St

12th Ave E

14th Ave E

E Republican St

E Harrison St

13th Ave E

16th Ave E

E Harrison St

E Thomas St

E Thomas St

Broadway E

E John St

Group Health
Capitol Hill
Campus
St Nicholas
Russian Orthodox
Cathedral

E Denny Way

E Denny Way

E Madison St

| 0 | 400 | 800 | 1,200 yards |
| 0 | 400 | 800 | 1,200 meters |

E Howell St

finish

E Olive St

24 east capitol Hill: MILLIONaires' row and pioneer graves

BOUNDARIES: 13th Ave. E., E. Olive St., 16th Ave E., and E. Howe St.
DISTANCE: 2¾ miles
DIFFICULTY: Easy (almost all flat)
PARKING: Free street parking
PUBLIC TRANSIT: Metro route #10 stops near this walk's start.

Seattle used to be promoted as having "seven hills," just like Rome. We lost one of those to the Denny Regrade (Walk 5). Of the remaining slopes, only one is known simply as "The Hill." It's Capitol Hill, rising just east of downtown. For decades it was Seattle's densest neighborhood, before all the Belltown condo towers went up. It's still a hearty mélange of students, artists, gays, families, and folks of many subcultures and ethnicities. Our next three walks traverse different portions of The Hill. This particular walk takes you to its summit, and includes a regal cemetery, a palatial greenhouse, an art deco museum housing Asian art, some huge old mansions, and some solid old middle-class homes and apartments.

- Start on 15th Ave. E. and E. Garfield St., at Louisa Boren Park. It's a tall bluff above, and connected to, Interlaken Park (Walk 23). From here you can also see Lake Washington, the Cascade mountains, and Bellevue. Turn south onto 15th, then walk briefly southeast on 15th to Lake View Cemetery's entrance. It's got the remains of some of Seattle's founding families (some of whom were moved up to three times, as early burial lands were redeveloped).

- Take a clockwise loop through the cemetery's paved paths, as follows:

  Go straight from the entrance until the path bends left.

  Take the first right. As this path curves south, to your right you see the elaborate monument to sawmill baron Henry Yesler, his wife, and an unnamed third person (rumored to be the female lover of either or both Yeslers). Just beyond that is the far plainer gravestone of Princess Angeline, daughter of Chief Sealth (for whom Seattle's named).

Follow this curving perimeter path around the property's west and then north sides. Elaborate Victorian monuments bear family names you've already seen on your walks—Chittenden, Mercer, Bell, Stone, Nordstrom—while smaller markers remember hundreds of the more obscure. This path curves south near the Nisei Monument, honoring Japanese Americans who died in World War II.

Turn right at a four-way crossroads; then turn left. Winding southeast from a mausoleum, you find the Denny family's quite elaborate monument. Across the road from that are Lake View's most famous graves, those of actor Bruce Lee and his son Brandon. Due south of there, a big sequoia tree stands above the very modest grave markers of David "Doc" Maynard and his wife Catherine (Walk 33).

Take two left turns and one right turn, back to the entrance gate and to 15th.

● Turn south on 15th, which at this point has a sidewalk only on its east side. Cross back to the west side at the

Back Story: The Olmsted Plan

In 1903, Seattle hired the Massachusetts-based Olmsted Brothers design firm to devise a master plan for the city's park system. The Olmsteds (whose father, Frederick Law Olmsted, had designed New York City's Central Park) came up with a scheme to place a park or playground within a half mile of every home in town, connected by 20 miles of broad boulevards with wide green median strips. Led by John Charles and Frederick Law, Jr., the Olmsted firm continued to consult on Seattle's open spaces for the next three decades.

intersection with E. Galer St., which becomes E. Highland Dr. as it enters Volunteer Park.

- Walk southwest along Highland past a kids' play area, toward the statue of Alaska Purchase instigator William Seward. Behind that is the Volunteer Park Conservatory, a Victorian greenhouse styled after London's Crystal Palace. Its five main rooms house cacti, ferns, palms, bromeliads (members of the pineapple family), and seasonally-rotated plant displays.

- Turn south from the statue on Volunteer Park Rd. To your left is the Seattle Asian Art Museum, whose 1933 Art Moderne building is as beautiful as any of the works within it. To your right, Isamu Noguchi's circular sculpture *Black Sun* (inspiration for the Soundgarden song title) frames a Space Needle view, with a large reservoir in between. Ahead of you is a 75-foot-tall water tower. If you climb its 106 steps, you reach an observation deck with great views and educational posters about the Olmsted Brothers' park plan.

- From the tower's south side, leave the park heading south on 14th Ave. E. You're on "Millionaires' Row," a largely intact strip of opulent, large early-20th-century homes. One of them, the Shafer Baillie Mansion at 14th and Aloha, is now a bed-and-breakfast.

- Turn east on E. Roy St., the old southern end to Millionaires' Row. (Its homeowners once had a gate installed here, even though it's a public street.) When you're back at 15th, turn right. This is more typical Capitol Hill housing stock—some Classic Box houses, some Craftsman bungalows, and some early- to mid-20th century apartments.

South of E. Mercer St. are the quasi-Tudor Fredonia Apartments, with the classically unpretentious Canterbury Ale & Eats on the ground floor. This is start of the 15th Ave. business strip. These four packed blocks mix the basics (a drugstore, regular and "natural" groceries, and a dry cleaners) with gift boutiques, coffeehouses, and many kinds of bars and restaurants. Of particular note are European Vine Selections (a wine shop with a plain storefront and a huge selection), Coastal Kitchen (an upscale fish house), and Victrola Coffee and Art (a coffeehouse always packed with local characters).

- Turn east on E. Thomas St. for one block. To your south is the main campus of Group Health Cooperative, founded in 1947 as a patient-owned health care provider. Today it's one of the big five "Pill Hill" medical complexes on Capitol and First hills.

- Turn south on 16th Ave. E. for three blocks, past modest prewar homes and classic brick apartments. At the corner with E. John St., a distinguished-looking former Methodist church now houses an Internet marketing firm. A block away at E. Denny Way, an equally handsome former Christian Science church has been divided into condos.

- Head west on E. Howell St. for three blocks. At 15th and Howell, the Gaslight Inn B&B occupies a particularly fancy old bungalow. At 13th, the Greek Orthodox Church of the Assumption is a clean white '60s structure topped by a modern, modest dome that's best seen from the back.

- Turn south one block on 13th to view the smaller but much more elaborate Saint Nicholas Russian Orthodox Cathedral. Its roof features three golden onion domes surrounding a six-sided spire. On the block's end at E. Olive St. is the Advent Christian Church, a solid brick box.

- From here you can return east to 15th, or continue south one more block to E. Pine St. Either option will lead to a #10 bus heading back to your start.

CONNECTING THE WALKS

This walk connects easily to two other walks. At 13th and Aloha you're three blocks east of Walk 25. This route ends one block north of Walk 26.

POINTS OF INTEREST

Lake View Cemetery lakeviewcemeteryassociation.com, 1554 15th Ave. E., 206-322-1582

Volunteer Park Conservatory volunteerparkconservatory.org, 1402 E. Galer St., 206-322-4112

Seattle Asian Art Museum seattleartmuseum.org, 1400 E. Prospect St., 206-654-3100

Shafer Baillie Mansion sbmansion.com, 907 14th Ave. E., 206-322-4654

Canterbury Ale & Eats 534 15th Ave. E., 206-322-3130

European Vine Selections evswines.com, 522 15th Ave E., 206-323-3557

Victrola Coffee and Art victrolacoffee.com, 411 15th Ave. E., 206-325-6520

Group Health Capitol Hill Campus ghc.org, 201 16th Ave. E.

St. Nicholas Russian Orthodox Cathedral saintnicholascathedral.org, 1714 13th Ave. E., 206-322-9387

route summary

1. Start on 15th Ave. E., walking south from E. Garfield St. to Lake View Cemetery.
2. Take a clockwise loop route through the cemetery, and back to 15th.
3. Turn south on 15th.
4. Turn southeast on E. Highland Dr. into Volunteer Park.
5. Turn south on Volunteer Park Rd. to the water tower. Walk around to the water tower's south side.
6. Leave the park, going south on 14th Ave. E.
7. Turn east on E. Roy St.
8. Turn south on 15th Ave. E.
9. Turn east on E. Thomas St.
10. Turn south on 16th Ave. E.
11. Turn west on E. Howell St.
12. Turn south on 13th Ave. to E. Olive St.

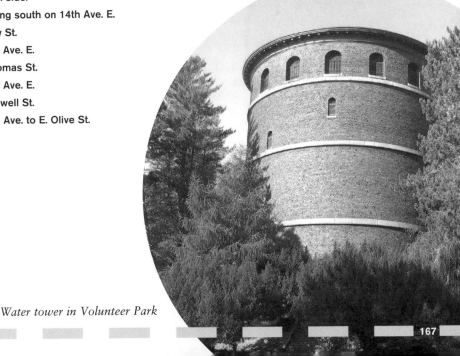

Water tower in Volunteer Park

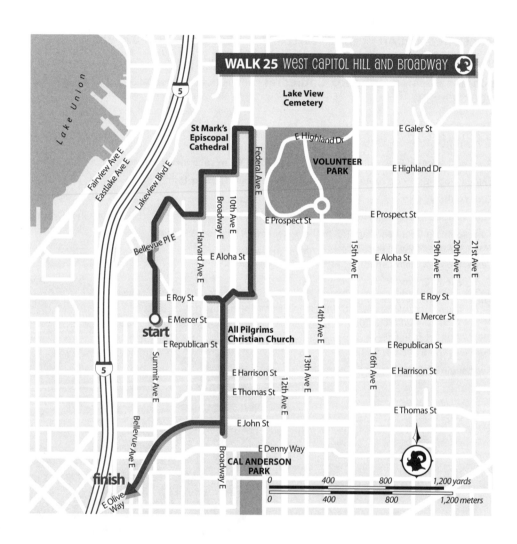

Lake Union

5

Lake View Cemetery

St Mark's Episcopal Cathedral

E Galer St

E Highland Dr

VOLUNTEER PARK

E Highland Dr

Fairview Ave E

Eastlake Ave E

Lakeview Blvd E

Federal Ave E

10th Ave E

Broadway E

E Prospect St

E Prospect St

15th Ave E

19th Ave E

20th Ave E

21st Ave E

Bellevue Pl E

Harvard Ave E

E Aloha St

E Aloha St

16th Ave E

E Roy St

E Roy St

start

E Mercer St

E Mercer St

E Republican St

All Pilgrims Christian Church

14th Ave E

E Republican St

Summit Ave E

E Harrison St

13th Ave E

E Harrison St

E Thomas St

12th Ave E

E Thomas St

E John St

Bellevue Ave E

E Denny Way

Broadway E

CAL ANDERSON PARK

finish

E Olive Way

| 0 | 400 | 800 | 1,200 yards |
| 0 | 400 | 800 | 1,200 meters |

25 WEST CAPITOL HILL AND BROADWAY: BROADWAY BOUND

BOUNDARIES: **Federal Ave. E., E. Galer St., Bellevue Ave. E., and E. Olive Way**
DISTANCE: **2¼ miles**
DIFFICULTY: **Moderate (two modest inclines)**
PARKING: **Free street parking**
PUBLIC TRANSIT: **Metro route #14 stops at this walk's start.**

This walk reveals The Hill in all its multivalent, diverse glory. And along the way you'll see some great architecture, including a monumental and deliberately unfinished Episcopalian church, some more sumptuous old-money mansions, and the eccentric masterworks of a highly individualistic apartment designer. You end up on Broadway, The Hill's traditional main drag. While the street's undergone a lot of changes and revamps in recent years, it remains a vital eating, shopping, and people-watching corridor.

● Start on the northwest corner of Summit Ave. E. and E. Mercer St. in front of a couple of local hangout bars and the handsomely decked-out original location of Top Pot Doughnuts. Head north on Summit for two blocks, past some Classic Box houses and unpretentious low-rise apartments.

This stretch of Summit ends at Belmont Ave. E. In front of you is one of the idiosyncratic apartment buildings designed and built in the 1920s by self-taught architect Frederick Anhalt. His projects are known for Tudor- and Norman-inspired design flourishes and for central courtyards, bestowing a sense of community. Cross Belmont for a better view of this and another Anhalt building to its right.

● Dogleg northwest briefly on Belmont, north on another brief piece of Summit, northeast very briefly on Bellevue Pl. E., then north again on yet another segment of Summit. This area is part of the Harvard-Belmont Landmark District, full of large, well-preserved old homes. One particular highlight is the relatively small Bower/Bystrom House, a blue-and-white gingerbread cottage above a street-level garage.

- Continue as Summit bends northeast. This stretch is a narrow road with big curbside trees in front of even bigger prewar houses.

- Summit becomes E. Prospect St, bending southeast. As you round this corner you see the back of the O. W. Fisher and O. D. Fisher houses. These exquisite Tudor manses were built for the flour-milling family whose descendants own KOMO-TV (Walk 5). A closer view can be had as you pass the intersection with Belmont Pl. E.

- Prospect turns east (and slightly uphill) at the next intersection. To your left is a brick wall marking the original southern boundary of Horace C. Henry's estate. He was the railroad baron who funded the UW's Henry Art Gallery (Walk 19).

- Turn north on Harvard Ave. E. To your left, you see more of the former Henry property behind a hedge. But you won't see Henry's mansion; it was razed in 1937. Farther up the street to your right, the new Harvard & Highland condo buildings try to fit in with their surroundings with a surfeit of "luxury" details.

- At Harvard's end, turn east onto E. Highland Dr. To your left is the hulking 1910 concrete mansion of Sam Hill, part of the family that owned the Great Northern Railway. He also commissioned the Maryhill Museum and Stonehenge replica in southwest Washington and the Peace Arch at the Canadian border near Interstate 5.

- Turn north on 10th Ave. E. To your right is the tasteful brick A-frame structure of Trinity Lutheran Church. A grander religious statement awaits on the left side of 10th. It's the "holy box" of St. Mark's Episcopal Cathedral. Designed in 1930 as a neo-Byzantine palace of worship, Depression-era finances left it unfinished, particularly on the outside. Some brick cladding was finally stuck onto the front decades later. Behind the building, a preserved greenbelt with a privately maintained garden extends down the Hill's northwest slope. To its north, the Gage Academy of Art occupies a former girls' school that was later part of Cornish College (Walk 6).

- Turn east on E. Galer St. On your right is an elaborate stucco mansion known among neighbors as "the Pink Palace." It was built in 1910 by Henry Kleinberg, a successful hay merchant. It was up for sale in 2010 for a mere $4.8 million. To your left is a brick Tudor mansion once owned by KING-TV founder Dorothy Bullitt.

● Turn south on Federal Ave. E. for four blocks. Most of the homes here are of more modest, upper-middle-class size, but still handsome and well-kept. It's hard to believe much of Capitol Hill was once in steep decline. In the 1970s, the "Boeing Bust" recession combined with white flight and suburbanization to send neighborhood housing prices into a tailspin. They soared back and then some in the 1990s and 2000s, then dipped a little again.

● Turn west on E. Roy St., between two more classic Anhalt apartment buildings. In the 1980s, the building on the south side was the fictional home of comic book hero Green Arrow. Continue as Roy bends southwest to Broadway E.

On the southeast side of Broadway and Roy is the Deluxe Bar & Grill, a neighborhood hangout since the 1930s. To its west, the stately Women's Century Club has housed the Harvard Exit, a leading art-house cinema, since the 1970s. Across Roy from that is a Daughters of the American Revolution chapter, designed as a small-scale replica of George Washington's Mount Vernon, New York, home. East of that is the Loveless Building, a 1930 apartment-retail structure. It's another Tudor Revival affair, complete with a central courtyard. One tenant, the Olivar restaurant, has an elaborate mural depicting a Pushkin fairy tale. It's left over from the Russian restaurant originally in that space.

● Return to the east side of Broadway. Two blocks (and two block-long mixed-use megaprojects) later, All Pilgrims Christian Church is a century-old brick edifice with great acoustics inside and a gay-friendly rainbow flag outside.

● Continue south through the Broadway retail strip. Here are trendy bistros (Broadway Grill, Julia's, Bleu), untrendy bars (Charlie's), affordable ethnic meals (Jai Thai, Pho Cyclo), espresso joints (Vivace, Dilletante), clothes (Red Light, Metro Clothing), and much more. Kitty-corner from All Pilgrims is the Broadway Market building. The 1989 complex preserves the name, and the brick-and-terra-cotta facade, of a 1928 mini-mall. There's another false front at Broadway and E. Olive Way, where a Rite Aid pharmacy sits behind the old Broadway Theater's marquee. Halfway down the next block is another Dick's Drive-In. Its walk-up windows host an ever-changing human parade.

- Turn west on Olive, which soon curves southwest. Here are more cool eateries (B&O Espresso, Dinette), bars (Stumbling Monk, Captain Black's, the Living Room, Faire), and shops (including the Pretty Parlor retro-fashion boutique). At Olive and Bellevue Ave. E., City Market is an indie deli-mart with cute cartoon sandwich signs in front, often in the form of ersatz celebrity endorsements.

- From here you can backtrack to Olive and Howell, and catch a #14 bus to your starting point. Or you can backtrack a little farther to Olive and Summit, then walk five blocks north back to Mercer.

CONNECTING THE WALKS

This walk connects easily to four other walks. From St. Mark's you can take a steep downhill trail to Walk 23. At Federal and E. Aloha St. you're four blocks west of Walk 24. At Federal and 10th you're three-quarters of a mile south of Walk 23. At E. Olive Way and E. Denny Way you're three steep downhill blocks east of Walk 6. This walk ends two blocks north of Walk 26.

POINTS OF INTEREST

Top Pot Doughnuts toppotdoughnuts.com, 609 Summit Ave. E., 206-323-7841

St. Mark's Episcopal Cathedral saintmarks.org, 1245 10th Ave. E., 206-323-0300

Anhalt Apartments 1005 E. Roy St.

Harvard Exit Theater landmarktheatres.com, 807 E. Roy St., 206-781-5755

All Pilgrims Christian Church allpilgrims.org, 500 Broadway E., 206-322-0487

B&O Espresso b-oespresso.com, 204 Belmont Ave. E., 206-322-5028

Pretty Parlor prettyparlor.com, 110 Summit Ave. E., 206-405-2883

City Market 1722 Bellevue Ave., 206-323-1715

route summary

1. Start on Summit Ave. E., walking north from E. Mercer St.
2. Dogleg northwest briefly on Belmont Ave. E., north briefly on Summit, northeast briefly on Bellevue Pl. E., then north again on Summit.
3. Continue as Summit bends northeast.
4. Continue as Summit becomes E. Prospect St, bending southeast, then east.
5. Turn north on Harvard Ave. E.
6. Turn east on E. Highland Dr.
7. Turn north on 10th Ave. E.
8. Turn east on E. Galer St.
9. Turn south on Federal Ave. E.
10. Turn west on E. Roy St., which bends southwest.
11. Turn south on Broadway E.
12. Turn west on E. Olive Way, curving southwest to Bellevue Ave. E.

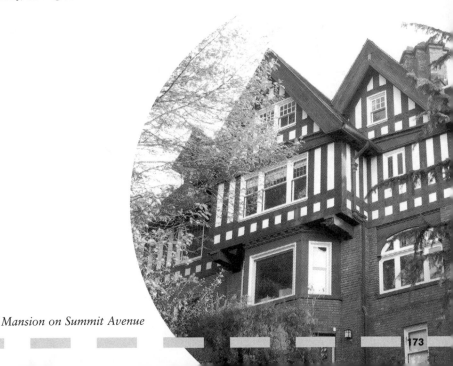

Mansion on Summit Avenue

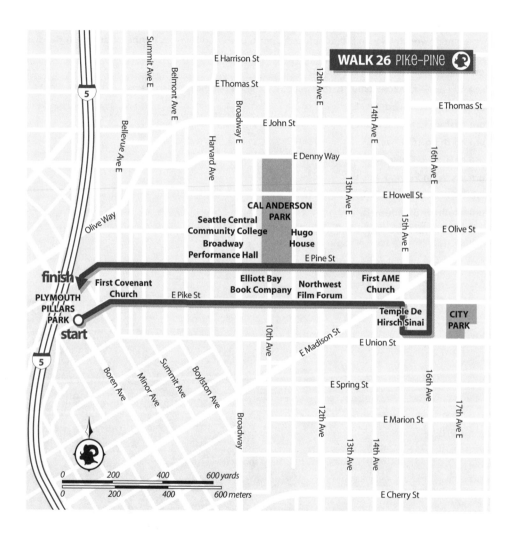

E Harrison St

E Thomas St

Summit Ave E

Belmont Ave E

Broadway E

Bellevue Ave E

Harvard Ave

12th Ave E

14th Ave E

E Thomas St

E John St

16th Ave E

E Denny Way

13th Ave E

E Howell St

E Olive St

15th Ave E

Olive Way

CAL ANDERSON PARK

Seattle Central Community College

Broadway Performance Hall

Hugo House

E Pine St

finish

PLYMOUTH PILLARS PARK

start

First Covenant Church

E Pike St

Elliott Bay Book Company

Northwest Film Forum

First AME Church

Temple De Hirsch Sinai

CITY PARK

10th Ave

E Madison St

E Union St

16th Ave

17th Ave E

Boren Ave

Minor Ave

Summit Ave

Boylston Ave

Broadway

E Spring St

12th Ave

13th Ave

14th Ave

E Marion St

E Cherry St

0   200   400   600 yards

0   200   400   600 meters

26 PIKE-PINE: alternative Ground Zero

BOUNDARIES: **Boren Ave., E. Pike St., 16th Ave. E., and E. Pine St.**
DISTANCE: **2 miles**
DIFFICULTY: **Moderate (half gently uphill, half gently downhill)**
PARKING: **Metered street parking; a pay lot on Pike east of Boren**
PUBLIC TRANSIT: **Metro routes #10, 11, 14, 43, and 49 stop at this walk's start.**

Broadway's dominance of the Capitol Hill business scene has been supplanted in recent years by the Pike-Pine Corridor. Once Seattle's Auto Row, its handsome prewar showrooms and garages now house the bulk of The Hill's gay, music, art, and theater scenes; plus still more places at which to eat, drink, and shop. (As with many of this book's walks, there are far too many cool spaces to mention in these pages; take the time to make your own discoveries.) Along the way, this walk passes a major indie bookstore in a former auto-parts warehouse, a ballroom dance studio in a former Odd Fellows hall, a literary arts center in a former funeral parlor, and two separate quartets of Greek-style architectural columns, disembodied from the houses of worship they once fronted.

● Start at Plymouth Pillars Park, at the northwest corner of Pike St. and Boren Ave. It overlooks Interstate 5, the downtown skyline, Queen Anne Hill, and the Space Needle. The titular columns are from the original Plymouth Congregational Church (Walk 3), razed to make way for I-5.

● Walk northeast on Pike, which bends east one block later. The architectural aesthetic is more prewar-industrial, less ostentatious, than the previous two Capitol Hill walks. You're on Seattle's original "Auto Row." One surviving car dealership, Seattle Volvo, exists just beyond Boren. Other ex-showroom and garage buildings now host hangout restaurants (Six Arms), gay bars (Seattle Eagle), and stores (Utrecht Art Supplies). East of Bellevue Ave. E., First Covenant Church features a circular sanctuary under a gilt-tipped dome. The century-old congregation was originally founded by Swedish immigrants.

Another still-extant car seller, Phil Smart Mercedes, sports an appropriately understated storefront at Pike and Boylston St. Kitty-corner from there stands a three-story bay-windowed apartment complex; its street-level shops include the nationally famous sex-toy store Babeland. Beyond Pike and Harvard, the recently built Harvard Market retail complex on your right tries to fit in with the old two-story brick structures on your left.

● Continue on Pike east of Broadway, through the beating heart of Seattle's art-hipster realm. Amid the poster-encrusted light poles and strewn copies of *The Stranger* newspaper, you may find the coffee crowd (Caffe Vita), the beer crowd (Comet Tavern, Elysian Brewpub), the cocktail crowd (Quinn's, Bimbo's Cantina), the cheap-eats crowd (Ballet, Piecora's Pizza), the live-rock crowd (Neumo's, Chop Suey), the live-theater crowd (Annex, Bagalan, Velocity Dance), the gay male crowd (The Unicorn), and the gay female crowd (the Wild Rose, Washington's only official lesbian bar).

The side streets here have their own attractions. North of Pike on 10th Ave. is the Elliott Bay Book Co., a wooden-shelved cathedral of literary mellowness recently moved from Pioneer Square. North of Pike at 11th are more hip bars, plus the acclaimed Vermillion Gallery and the Crypt fetish-wear shop. North of Pike on 12th is the Northwest Film Forum, a year-round film festival and film school in one.

● Turn south on 15th Ave. from a long, low roadhouse structure (once the C. C. Attle's gay bar). To your left is the full-block campus of Temple De Hirsch Sinai, Seattle's principal Jewish congregation. At the end of the block, north of Union St., is a small park atop a short set of steps, with another quartet of building columns. They're from the temple's original building, razed in 1993. Walk through the park and the parking lot behind it, to 16th Ave. You can now see the temple's 1960-built Alhadeff Sanctuary with its fez-like, 14-sided dome.

● Turn north on 16th to the six-way intersection with E. Madison St. and E. Pine St. The big Beaux Arts building to your right is the Olympian Apartments seen in the films *House of Games* and *The Fabulous Baker Boys*. On Madison's west side is Madison Market, a natural foods co-op.

● Turn west on Pine. You pass some bubble-era mixed-use behemoths. Then at the southeast corner of 14th and Pine is the First AME Church, Seattle's biggest historically black congregation. At 13th Ave., the Cuff Complex's tiny sign is a throwback to when gay bars had to look inconspicuous. At 11th Ave., Cal Anderson Park is one of the city's most used active-recreation parks; it was recently enlarged by covering an adjacent reservoir.

Just north of Pine on 11th, Richard Hugo House is a literary arts center in an old funeral home. At 10th, the venerable Odd Fellows Hall used to have a lot of theater and dance troupes in its once-cheap spaces. It still has the Century Ballroom inside (lindy hop lessons weekly) and a swank yet homey bistro and bar outside.

At Pine and Broadway, an art supply store occupies a lavish former Pontiac dealership. In front of the store is a kitschy life-size statue of Jimi Hendrix, installed when an office-music company occupied the building. Across Broadway is Seattle Central Community College. It's won awards for its programs but not for its architecture, a slab of '70s brutalism that replaced the grand Edwardian Broadway High School. Broadway High's auditorium annex survives as the Broadway Performance Hall, host to dance and theater events.

Across Pine, SCCC has expanded into a former Masonic Temple. That building's main auditorium is leased to the Egyptian Theatre; every May it's ground zero for the Seattle International Film Festival (the biggest event of its kind in the United States).

On Pine west of Harvard Ave., Bill's Off Broadway Pizza starts another stretch of booze joints (Linda's, Capitol Club, R Place, Chapel), snack joints (Hot Mama's Pizza, 611 Supreme Crepes), and caffeine joints (the cool and classy Bauhaus Books & Coffee). There's unique shopping here too—Asian and Indian gifts, retro-modern furniture, young fashions, and rare LPs.

● Pine bends southwest at Melrose Ave., by the posh dance club The Baltic Room. Just beyond Minor Ave., take a left turn back into Plymouth Pillars Park. This section has an off-leash dog park space, and some oversize concrete urns from the old Music Hall theater downtown (demolished in 1992). You're just across Boren from your start.

CONNECTING THE WALKS

This walk connects easily to a half dozen other walks. It starts and ends across the Interstate 5 overpass from Walks 2 and 3. At Broadway and Pike you're one block north of Walk 27. At 16th and Union you're two blocks west of Walk 28. At 13th and Pine you're one block south of Walk 24. At Bellevue and Pine you're two blocks south of Walk 25.

POINTS OF INTEREST

Plymouth Pillars Park seattle.gov/parks, Boren Ave. and Pike St.

First Covenant Church firstcovenantseattle.org, 400 E. Pike St., 206-322-7411

Elliott Bay Book Co. elliottbaybook.com, 1521 10th Ave., 206-624-6600

Northwest Film Forum nwfilmforum.org, 1515 12th Ave., 206-329-2629

Temple De Hirsch Sinai tdhs-nw.org, 1511 E. Pike St., 206-323-8486

First AME Church fameseattle.org, 1522 14th Ave., 206-324-3664

Richard Hugo House hugohouse.org, 1634 11th Ave., 206-322-7030

Seattle Central Community College seattlecentral.edu, 1701 Broadway, 206-587-3800

Broadway Performance Hall broadwayperfhall.com, 1625 Broadway, 206-325-3113

Egyptian Theatre landmarktheatres.com, 805 E. Pine St., 206-720-4560

route summary

1. Start on Pike St., walking northeast from Boren Ave. Pike bends east one block later.

2. Turn south on 15th Ave.

3. Cut through the park north of 15th and Union St., to 16th Ave.

4. Turn north on 16th to the six-way with E. Madison St. and E. Pine St.

5. Turn west on E. Pine St.

6. Turn southwest at Minor Ave. into Plymouth Pillars Park, then walk through the park back to Pike and Boren.

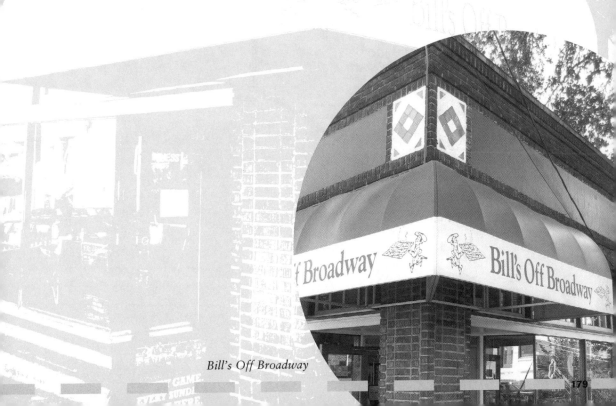

Bill's Off Broadway

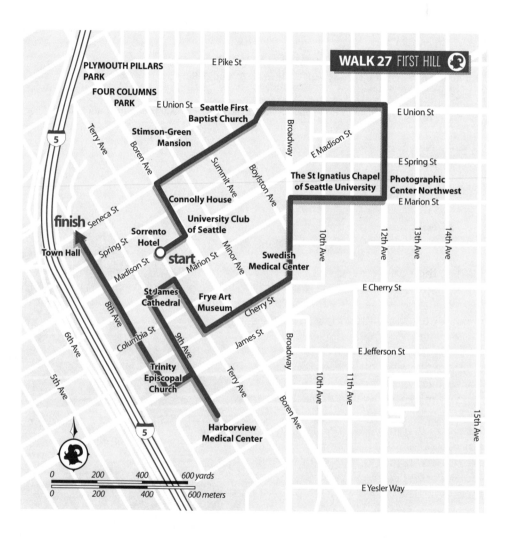

PLYMOUTH PILLARS
PARK

FOUR COLUMNS
PARK

E Pike St

E Union St

Seattle First
Baptist Church

E Union St

Stimson-Green
Mansion

Broadway

E Madison St

E Spring St

Terry Ave

Boren Ave

Summit Ave

Boylston Ave

The St Ignatius Chapel
of Seattle University

Photographic
Center Northwest

Connolly House

E Marion St

University Club
of Seattle

12th Ave

13th Ave

14th Ave

finish

Seneca St

Sorrento
Hotel

10th Ave

Town Hall

Spring St

Madison St

start

Marion St

Minor Ave

Swedish
Medical Center

E Cherry St

8th Ave

St James
Cathedral

Frye Art
Museum

Cherry St

Columbia St

9th Ave

James St

Broadway

E Jefferson St

6th Ave

Trinity
Episcopal
Church

Terry Ave

10th Ave

11th Ave

5th Ave

5

Harborview
Medical Center

Boren Ave

15th Ave

0   200   400   600 yards

0   200   400   600 meters

E Yesler Way

5

27 FIRST HILL: PILLS, Prayers, and Paintings

BOUNDARIES: 12th Ave., Seneca St., 8th Ave., and E. Union St.
DISTANCE: 2¼ miles
DIFFICULTY: Moderate (mostly flat or downhill)
PARKING: Metered street parking; a pay lot
PUBLIC TRANSIT: Metro routes #2, 12, 60, and 64 stop near this walk's start.

"Seattle's 1st Neighborhood," as promotional street banners call it, is a residential neighborhood overlooking downtown. Once the timber came down from these slopes in the late 19th century, prestigious big homes went up; four of them are still standing as restored historic sites. It's also informally known as "Pill Hill," with most of Seattle's major hospitals, and as "Catholic Hill," with several major ecclesiastical institutions including the city's principal cathedral, a Jesuit university campus, and an angular modern chapel. You also pass art spaces devoted to realist painting and contemporary photography, and a stunning century-old hotel.

- Start at the northwest corner of Terry Ave. and Madison St., just outside the Sorrento Hotel's grand courtyard. The grand Italian villa–style boutique hotel is another legacy from the 1909 Alaska-Yukon-Pacific Exposition (Walk 19). If you have the time, peek inside at the sumptuous lobby and Fireside Room.

- Head northeast on Madison for one block. To your left are two old, terra-cotta clad, single-story retail buildings. To your right is a bubble-era mixed-use behemoth. At Boren Ave., the University Club of Seattle occupies a grand old turn-of-the-last-century mansion, behind some thick shrubbery.

- Turn northwest onto Boren Ave. and continue for two blocks. To your left, the Hide-out is a dark, tastefully signed storefront bar that's become a hangout for the local art scene. To your right at Boren and Spring, the William Hofius House (a 1902 foursquare-style mansion) is now Connolly House, headquarters to the Catholic archbishop of Seattle.

- Turn northeast on Seneca St. and continue for four blocks. Among this stretch's elegant old apartment buildings are two more vintage mansions. The 1907 Dearborn

House, at the southwest corner of Seneca and Minor Ave., is now home to the preservation group Historic Seattle. Kitty-corner from there, the 1899 Stimson-Green Mansion is owned by another nonprofit, the Washington Trust for Historic Preservation and is a popular wedding and party site.

- At the five-way intersection of Seneca, Harvard Ave., and Union St., see the noble Seattle First Baptist Church (built in stages from 1910 to 1920), with its gentle juxtaposition of curves and angles. Dogleg left along Harvard toward Union, at a dark brick Knights of Columbus hall.

- Turn east on Union, the cusp between the First Hill and Capitol Hill neighborhoods. Gilda's Club, part of a circuit of cancer-support centers named for comedienne Gilda Radner, sits at Broadway and Union. The former law-office building's front replicates the front of Thomas Jefferson's home in Monticello, Virginia. Looking south from there, Garage is a bar and pool hall that's also got some of Seattle's last public bowling lanes.

  On the southeast side of 10th Ave. and Union, a weathered old commercial building juxtaposes an auto-repair shop with an art gallery, a tattoo parlor, and a fringe-theater studio. Directly east of that building is Po Dog (a hipster hot dog joint). Looking south of Union on 10th, you can glimpse Seattle's last blue-roofed IHOP restaurant. At 11th Ave. and Union, the Lifelong AIDS Alliance runs a fashionable thrift store.

- At the six-way intersection of Union, 12th Ave., and Madison St. are two extremes in contemporary nightlife—Tavern Law, a very inconspicuous neo-speakeasy, and Pony, a very visible gay dance club. Turn south on 12th, past the Seattle Academy of Arts and Sciences (a private secondary school), Cafe Presse (a soccer bar and espresso joint), and Photographic Center Northwest (where members and students still take pictures with film).

- Turn west on E. Marion St. and walk through the Seattle University campus. One block into the grounds, turn to your right to see a reflecting pool in front of the Chapel of St. Ignatius. The Jesuit university's first on-campus church is a meditative masterwork of light, color, and juxtaposed shapes, as designed in the 1990s by architect

Steven Holl. Many critics compare it favorably to another local work of postmodern asymmetry, the Experience Music Project (Walk 5).

Continue westward through SU, past a pleasant mix of 1920s, 1960s, and 1990s structures. At this point, your path turns moderately uphill, including three short sets of stairs. Just before you leave the campus grounds at Broadway, you see a bust of Chief Seattle to your right.

● Turn south on Broadway. You soon see the grand entrance to Swedish Medical Center, the crown of Pill Hill. Cross Broadway at Columbia St. for a closer look at the gently curving white front of this massive health-care complex.

● Turn southwest on Cherry St., through the Swedish campus. Across Boren, you see banners promoting the Frye Art Museum. Continue to the Frye's main entrance at Terry Ave. and Cherry. Funded by the estate of meatpacking moguls Charles and Emma Frye, and originally dedicated to realist painting, it now hosts a variety of contemporary and classical exhibits. Even if you don't stop in (admission's always free), the front plaza's a pleasant spot to relax before resuming your journey.

● Turn northwest on Terry. You're soon flanked by the buildings of O'Dea High, a parochial boys' school founded in 1923. On your left as you approach Marion St., St. James Cathedral looks spectacular even from the back.

● Turn left on Marion and left again on 9th Ave., for a full view of St. James' exterior. The Italian Renaissance–style edifice originally opened in 1907; it's been revamped, inside and out, several times. Still here from the beginning are the grand staircase and the two square, 167-foot towers in front. The bronze doors were added in 1999. The interior is even more magnificent; tours are held weekly during summer.

Continue southeast on 9th. On your right south of Cherry, the German Heritage Society is ensconced in an 1885 US Assay Office, a two-story painted brick building with quaint old-west flourishes. Two blocks from there, Harborview Medical Center's 1931 institutional Art Deco has been compromised a bit with recent additions, including a six-story, glass-walled skybridge across 9th. South of the skybridge, the Moderne design motif remains, both in the main hospital to your right and in the Harborview Hall annex to your left (originally a nurses' dormitory).

- Backtrack on 9th to James St. and turn left, for one seriously downhill block. At 8th Ave. and James, the 1890 Trinity Episcopal Church is an English Gothic masterwork clad in rough stone.

- Turn northwest on 8th Ave. At Spring St., First Presbyterian is one of Seattle's oldest congregations (founded 1869) in a stunning midcentury modern edifice. Approaching Seneca St., Town Hall Seattle hosts lectures, panels, and recitals in a stucco-clad former Christian Science church (one of five reused Christian Science buildings described in this book). From here you're two uphill blocks away from Terry.

CONNECTING THE WALKS

This walk connects easily with four other walks. At 12th and Union you're one block south of Walk 26 and six blocks west of Walk 28. This walk ends one block northeast of Walk 3 and three blocks northeast of Walk 2.

POINTS OF INTEREST

Sorrento Hotel hotelsorrento.com, 900 Madison St., 206-343-6156

Stimson-Green Mansion stimsongreen.com, 1204 Minor Ave., 206-524-4918

Seattle First Baptist Church seattlefirstbaptist.org, 1111 Harvard Ave., 206-325-6051

Photographic Center Northwest pcnw.org, 900 12th Ave., 206-720-7222

Seattle University seattleu.edu, 901 12th Ave., 206-296-6000

Frye Art Museum fryemuseum.org, 704 Terry Ave., 206-622-9250

St. James Cathedral stjames-cathedral.org, 804 9th Ave., 206-622-3559

Trinity Episcopal Church trinityseattle.org, 609 8th Ave., 206-624-5337

Town Hall Seattle townhallseattle.org, 1119 8th Ave., 206-652-4255

route summary

1. Start on Madison St., walking northeast from Terry Ave.
2. Turn northwest on Boren Ave.
3. Turn northeast on Seneca St.
4. Turn left on Harvard Ave.
5. Turn east on E. Union St.
6. Turn south on 12th Ave.
7. Turn west on E. Marion St. Walk through the Seattle University campus.
8. Turn south on Broadway.
9. Turn southwest on Cherry St.
10. Turn northwest on Terry.
11. Turn southwest on Marion.
12. Turn southeast on 9th Ave.
13. Turn southwest on James St.
14. Turn northwest on 8th Ave. to Seneca St.

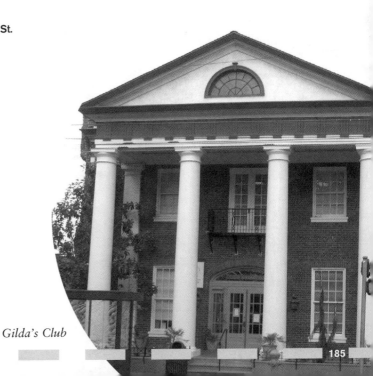

Gilda's Club

CITY PARK

E Madison St

E Union St

E Spring St

E Union St

E Spring St

Martin Luther King Jr Way

Immaculate Conception Church

E Marion St

E Columbia St

23rd Ave

24th Ave

13th Ave

14th Ave

16th Ave

12th Ave

E Cherry St

E Cherry St

Broadway

Swedish Medical Center: Cherry Hill Campus

E Jefferson St

Garfield High School

finish

start

10th Ave

11th Ave

Boren Ave

15th Ave

17th Ave

18th Ave

19th Ave

20th Ave

21st Ave

22nd Ave

E Alder St

E Spruce St

Washington Hall

Langston Hughes Performing Arts Center

E Fir St

25th Ave

26th Ave

27th Ave

Urban League of Metropolitan Seattle

E Yesler Way

EDWIN T PRATT PARK

Pratt Fine Arts Center

23rd Ave S

S Jackson St

12th Ave S

14th Ave S

16th Ave S

5

| 0 | 200 | 400 | 600 yards |
| 0 | 200 | 400 | 600 meters |

28 CENTRAL DISTRICT: SOUL CENTRAL

BOUNDARIES: 23rd Ave., E. Jackson St., 14th Ave., and E. Union St.
DISTANCE: 3 miles
DIFFICULTY: Moderate (mostly flat or downhill)
PARKING: Free and metered street parking
PUBLIC TRANSIT: Metro routes #3 and 4 stop at this walk's start.

This valley neighborhood, with no scenic views, was one of the few sections of Seattle where African Americans could own homes before the 1950s. It's still the spiritual center of the city's black community, even after the housing bubble displaced many longtime residents in favor of more upscale arrivistes. You'll see more humbly-sized, albeit handsomely preserved (in many cases), homes than in some of this book's other walks. The Central District also has its share of big institutional structures, including a theater in a former Jewish temple, another theater in a former Scandinavian community center, and a stoic brick formerly Catholic hospital.

- Start on the north side of E. Jefferson St., walking east from 17th Ave. You're in front of Swedish Medical Center: Cherry Hill Campus. The spire and neon cross atop this stately brick castle of medicine are left over from its original operators, the Sisters of Providence (in its day, the largest women-owned business in the state). A hospital-wide PA system used to play harp music to denote each newborn baby.

- Turn north on 18th Ave., initially along the hospital's back. At 18th and Columbia St. there's a tiny, plain, white-paneled storefront church. On the next block up is a more elaborate monument to faith, Immaculate Conception Catholic Church. The 1904 brick edifice is a mix of Romanesque, Baroque, and Byzantine design schticks, and features twin bell towers. Its many interior embellishments include a two-thirds scale replica of France's Our Lady of Lourdes Grotto.

- Across from T. T. Minor grade school at 18th and Union St. is a little strip of store-fronts, including the Gallery 1412 art and performance space. Turning east on the north side of Union, you soon reach Central Cinema, known for very eclectic programming. (Alongside artier fare, they once screened a "Worst of Madonna" film series.) Just north of Union on 22nd, Cappy's Boxing Gym is decorated with an exterior mural honoring "the sweet science."

● Turn south on 23rd Ave. past blocks of solid old homes, some of them recently remodeled with varying results. To your left south of E. Cherry St. is the sloped concrete facade of the Medgar Evers Pool, a public facility named for the Mississippi Civil Rights martyr. To your right at E. Jefferson St., Ezell's is a tiny fried-chicken joint that counts Oprah Winfrey among its fans. As you cross Jefferson, glance east to see the ex-Providence Hospital spire.

Continue south on 23rd, heading slightly uphill. On your left south of Jefferson, Garfield High School is a restored 1920s brick-and-terra-cotta masterpiece. Its high-profile alums include musicians Quincy Jones and Jimi Hendrix. At Yesler Way, the Douglass-Truth Library is a gracious old building (renamed in recent years after emancipation advocates Frederick Douglass and Sojourner Truth) combined with a sleek, metal-clad new building. Kitty-corner from there, the art deco Fire Station #6 features relief art of lightning bolts above its doors, symbolizing the then-new (1931) tool of radio dispatch. In more mundane modernity, a pair of strip malls, including a jazz-nostalgia themed Starbucks, stands at S. Jackson St.

● Turn west on Jackson. You soon pass Washington Middle School, the Washington Vocational Institute, the giant Franz bakery plant (its thrift store is a great spot for a mid-walk snack), several affordable Asian eateries, and, on a good day, a peep of Mt. Rainier to the southeast. At 18th Ave. S., the new Legacy Pratt Park apartment complex bears the restored rooftop sign of the block's former occupant, Wonder Bread. The bakery is gone, but the sign still leads motorists toward one of Seattle's least "whitebread" neighborhoods.

● Backtrack one block to 19th and Jackson; turn north. At 19th and S. Main St., the Pratt Fine Arts Center offers classes in sculpture, glass art, jewelry, and "2-D art." Tours are available by appointment. Continue north, into and through Edwin T. Pratt Park, to E. Yesler Way.

- Turn west on Yesler. At 17th Ave., the Langston Hughes Performing Arts Center has held theater, dance, film, and other events since 1969 in a majestic former synagogue. Appropriately, the building was designed in 1913 by B. Marcus Priteca, Seattle's foremost theater architect.

- Turn north on 14th Ave. at the old St. George Hotel. This stately Victorian brick edifice, with elegant brick-and-stone cladding, was built in 1910 as a residential hotel catering to Asian immigrants. It now houses the Urban League of Metropolitan Seattle. One block away at E. Fir St., Washington Hall was originally a 1908 Danish Brotherhood settlement house. It became a jazz venue in the 1940s, an African American Masonic lodge in the 1970s, and the original On the Boards performance space (Walk 8) in the 1980s. It still hosts theater and dance shows, under the management of preservation group Historic Seattle. Across 14th, the Squire Park P-Patch bears art panels by artist Mary Coss alongside the community garden plots.

- Continue on 14th for four blocks. To your left north of Spruce St., the King County Youth Center's public art (a tile mural, a whale-fin sculpture) fails to negate the sprawling, decaying '60s social-service complex's impersonal presence. A more human-scale presence awaits back at Jefferson St. in the form of Mesob, a mom-and-pop Ethiopian restaurant.

CONNECTING THE WALKS

This walk connects easily to two walks. It ends two blocks east and three blocks south of Walk 27. At 18th and Jackson you're six blocks east of Walk 11.

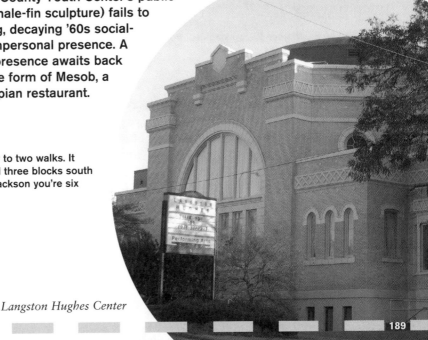

Langston Hughes Center

POINTS OF INTEREST

Swedish Medical Center: Cherry Hill Campus swedish.org, 500 17th Ave., 206-320-2000

Immaculate Conception Church immaculateconceptionseattle.org, 820 18th Ave., 206-322-5970

Central Cinema central-cinema.com, 1411 21st Ave., 206-686-6864

Ezell's Famous Chicken ezellschicken.com, 501 23rd Ave., 206-324-4141

Garfield High School ghs.seattleschools.org, 400 23rd Ave., 206-252-2270

Pratt Fine Arts Center pratt.org, 1902 S. Main St., 206-328-2200

Langston Hughes Performing Arts Center seattle.gov/parks/centers/Langston.htm, 104 17th Ave. S., 206-684-4758

Urban League of Metropolitan Seattle urbanleague.org, 105 14th Ave., 206-461-3792

Washington Hall washingtonhall.org, 153 14th Ave., 206-622-6952

ROUTE SUMMARY

1. Start on E. Jefferson St., walking east from 17th Ave.
2. Turn north on 18th Ave.
3. Turn east on E. Union St.
4. Turn south on 23rd Ave.
5. Turn west on S. Jackson St., to 18th Ave. S. Backtrack to 19th Ave. S.
6. Turn north on 19th. Walk through Edwin T. Pratt Park.
7. Turn west on E. Yesler Way.
8. Turn north on 14th Ave., back to Jefferson.

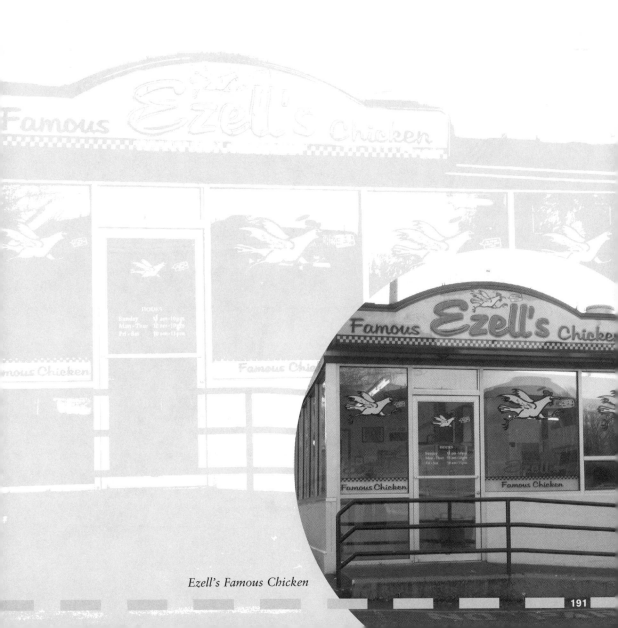

Ezell's Famous Chicken

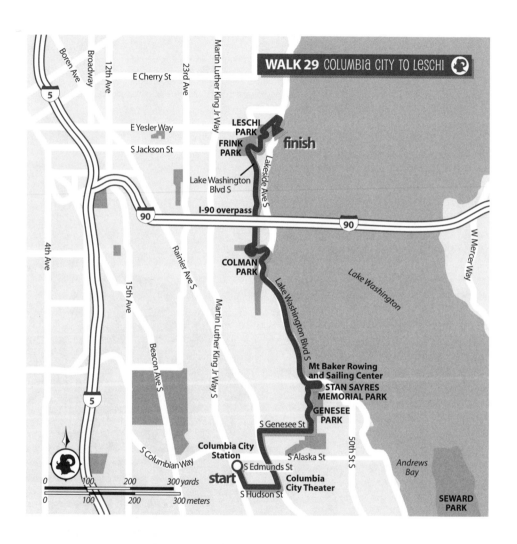

LESCHI PARK

FRINK PARK

finish

Lake Washington Blvd S

I-90 overpass

COLMAN PARK

Lakeside Ave S

Lake Washington Blvd S

Lake Washington

W Mercer Way

Mt Baker Rowing and Sailing Center

STAN SAYRES MEMORIAL PARK

GENESEE PARK

S Genesee St

50th St S

Columbia City Station

S Alaska St

Andrews Bay

S Edmunds St

start

Columbia City Theater

S Hudson St

SEWARD PARK

Boren Ave

Broadway

12th Ave

E Cherry St

23rd Ave

Martin Luther King Jr Way

E Yesler Way

S Jackson St

4th Ave

Rainier Ave S

15th Ave

Beacon Ave S

Martin Luther King Jr Way S

S Columbian Way

0   100   200   300 yards

0   100   200   300 meters

29 COLUMBIA CITY TO LESCHI: BETWEEN THE VALLEY AND THE "PITS"

BOUNDARIES: Martin Luther King Jr. Way S., S. Hudson St., Lake Washington Blvd.,
Lakeside Ave. S., and E. Yesler Way
DISTANCE: 5 miles
DIFFICULTY: Moderate (long, with some short uphill segments)
PARKING: Metered street parking at Rainier Ave. S.
PUBLIC TRANSIT: Link light rail stops at this walk's start; Metro routes #7, 8, 39, and 42 stop near it.

This winding amble through Seattle's southeast corner starts at the former independent town of Columbia City, now a thriving community of classic storefronts and well-preserved middle class homes. (Some people claim that it is the most diverse neighborhood in the United States.) You continue along the bucolic Lake Washington shoreline, getting a lot closer to the water than you did in Walk 21, then pass another stretch of magnificent water-view estates. Before you return to the lake, you get a glorious glimpse of one of the nation's most spectacular (and lowest) bridges, the modern-day successor to one of the first spans of its type in the world.

● Start at the Columbia City light rail station, Martin Luther King Jr. Way S. and S. Edmunds St. This part of the Central Link route is at ground level. The area surrounding the station is festooned with elaborate public art, including Victoria Fuller's *Global Garden Shovel* (a 35-foot-tall spade bearing relief images of varied flora). Walk southeast on King for two blocks, to S. Hudson St.

● Turn east on Hudson for three blocks, past a small strip mall and modest old homes. The larger house at the northwest corner of 37th Ave. E. and Hudson used to be Columbia City's town hall, when it was a separate town (1892–1907). At the northwest corner of Rainier Ave. S. and Hudson, social service agencies now occupy a 1926 Spanish revival–style police station. Across Rainier, the Tutta Bella artisan-pizza restaurant occupies a classic brick-box storefront.

● Turn northwest on the east side of Rainier, through the Columbia City business district. It's a compact string of classic charming buildings. North of Tutta Bella, the Columbia City Theater's deceptively tiny box-office storefront belies the grand restored concert and performance space behind it. North of it, a handsome old-west wood facade houses the Columbia City Alehouse.

Beyond that are three more blocks of handsome and intimate brick, wood, and concrete shop buildings. They contain a bakery, art galleries, hair salons, secondhand shops, clothing boutiques, an old-fashioned meat market, a single-screen cinema, and eateries ranging from BBQ to sushi.

On Rainier's west side north of S. Angeline St., Columbia Park's gently sloping "village green" spans the short distance between the Columbia City branch library (a stunning 1915 Georgian Revival edifice) and the Rainier Valley Cultural Center (yet *another* former Christian Science church, now used for performances, classes, and banquets).

Across S. Alaska St., the Columbia Funeral Home occupies a large bungalow behind a well-landscaped front garden. The business has been there since 1917. Before that, it was the childhood home of Leo Lassen, who grew up to be the beloved radio voice of minor league baseball's Seattle Rainiers. The team played a mile north of here, at the now-razed Sick's Stadium.

- Continue on Rainier two more blocks, then turn east on S. Genesee St. for eight blocks. Once you pass another pair of strip malls, you're in the sprawling, residential Rainier Valley. It's part of zip code 98118. Columnist Neal Pierce (citing Census Bureau documents) has called this the most ethnically diverse neighborhood in the United States. Whether it's *the* most diverse or not, these blocks definitely mix households of many races, classes, and faiths, within unpretentious homes of many styles.

- Beyond 43rd Ave. S., Genesee St. intersects Genesee Park. Turn north through this green, mostly flat park to its northern boundary at Lake Washington Blvd. S. Just across the street and along the lakeshore is Stan Sayres Memorial Park, popularly known as "The Pits." This series of short piers is home every August to the uniquely Seattle sport of hydroplane boat racing. Any true Seattleite will tell you how the old piston-powered "hydros" were so much more fun than the turbine-engine boats that race these days. This park's also the site of the Mt. Baker Rowing and Sailing Center, where you can learn the arts of motorless boating.

● Turn west on Lake Washington Blvd., bending northwest then north along the lake-shore. You stay on this street for the rest of this walk. The next mile of it will be along the shore, on a walking and jogging path just east of the vehicular road. As mentioned in Walks 10 and 20, the lake's surface was lowered several feet in the early 20th century. The city held on to this stretch of the new lakefront as a park. You'll see swimmers and sunbathers along this mile on warm days, and joggers by the score every day, along the big water, the big sky, and the small and big trees. A wall of trees and shrubbery west of the street helps hide civilization's intrusion.

● At its northern end, Lake Washington Boulevard Park sports an inland extension known as Colman Park. The street forks here. Take the left fork to continue on Lake Washington Blvd., switchbacking up through Colman Park. You're on a narrow, curving street within a tall tree canopy, offering great contrast between light and shadow. To your right as you leave the park, there's a small brown house. It was one of the last buildings designed by Victor Steinbrueck, the architect and UW professor who led the drive to save the Pike Place Market from redevelopment (Walk 4). Just north of that are some small, rustic cottages designed from 1910 through 1915 by another prominent local architect, Ellsworth Storey.

● Continue north on Lake Washington Blvd. into the Mt. Baker neighborhood. The streets here have lake views; the houses are big and fancy. Beyond S. Day St., there's a landscaped clearing where you can see how far from the lake you've come. You're overlooking the twin-span Lake Washington Floating Bridge, the 1989–1991 replacement for the original 1940 span, which sank in a windstorm after the new bridge's first span opened. A plaque here honors Lacey V. Murrow, the state transportation chief who supervised the original bridge's creation. (He was the brother of newscaster Edward R. Murrow.) If you descend some steps along the landscaped terrace, you can see the tunnel entrance that greeted travelers on the old bridge with the concrete-relief slogan CITY OF SEATTLE, PORTAL OF THE NORTH PACIFIC. That tunnel is now for walkers and bicyclists only.

- Return to Lake Washington Blvd., heading north past posh homes with posher front yards. North of S. Irving St., the road forks again; take the left fork. North of S. Dearborn St., you're back within parkland, specifically the adjoining Frink and Leschi parks. The street again becomes narrow and curvy, this time heading downhill.

- At the fork with S. Jackson St., stay on Lake Washington Blvd. You leave and reenter the park. As you leave the park a second time, you cross under a beautiful concrete underpass (arched on the bottom, angular on top).

- You're soon back at the lakeshore at Lakeside Blvd. S., along a small retail strip that includes a deli-mart, a bakery, a Daniel's steakhouse, and a commercial marina. To return to your start, take a right on Lakeside to a bus stop for a #27 to downtown. This bus takes a scenic switchback route up Lake Dell Ave. Transfer at Boren Ave. and Yesler Way to a southbound #9 back to Columbia City, or go downtown and hop on the light rail.

CONNECTING THE WALKS

This walk connects easily to two other walks. It ends three-quarters of a mile south of Walk 21. At Frink Park you're a half mile east of Walk 28.

POINTS OF INTEREST

Columbia City Station soundtransit.org, Martin Luther King Jr. Way S. and S. Edmunds St.

Columbia City Theater columbiacitytheater.com, 4918 Rainier Ave. S., 206-723-0088

Rainier Valley Cultural Center seedseattle.org/seedarts/rvcc.html, 3515 S. Alaska St., 206-725-7517

Columbia Funeral Home columbiafuneralhome.com, 4567 Rainier Ave. S., 206-722-1100

Mt. Baker Rowing and Sailing Center mbrsc.org, 3800 Lake Washington Blvd. S., 206-386-1913

Colman Park seattle.gov/parks, 1800 Lake Washington Blvd. S

I-90 Overpass and Bike Tunnel traillink.com/trail/the-i-90-trail.aspx, Lake Washington Blvd. S. at S. Day St.

Frink and Leschi Parks seattle.gov/parks, 398 Lake Washington Blvd. S.

Daniel's Restaurant Steakhouse and Bar schwartzbros.com/daniels.cfm,
200 Lake Washington Blvd., 206-329-4191

route summary

1.   Start on Martin Luther King Jr. Way S. walking southeast from S. Edmunds St.

2.   Turn east on S. Hudson St.

3.   Turn northwest on Rainier Ave. S.

4.   Turn east on S. Genesee St.

5.   Turn north through Genesee Park.

6.   Turn west on Lake Washington Blvd., bending northwest then north along the lakeshore.

7.   Continue on Lake Washington Blvd. winding through and out of Colman Park and past the I-90 tunnel.

8.   Continue on Lake Washington Blvd. winding through Frink and Leschi parks,
     back to the lakeshore at Lakeside Blvd. S.

Lake Washington Boulevard

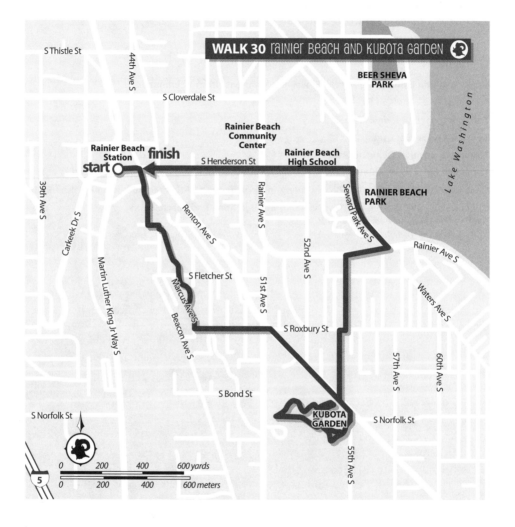

S Thistle St

44th Ave S

BEER SHEVA PARK

S Cloverdale St

Rainier Beach Community Center

Rainier Beach Station

finish

start

S Henderson St

Rainier Beach High School

RAINIER BEACH PARK

Lake Washington

39th Ave S

Carkeek Dr S

Renton Ave S

Rainier Ave S

Seward Park Ave S

52nd Ave S

Rainier Ave S

Martin Luther King Jr Way S

S Fletcher St

Marcus Ave S

51st Ave S

Beacon Ave S

S Roxbury St

Waters Ave S

57th Ave S

60th Ave S

S Bond St

KUBOTA GARDEN

S Norfolk St

55th Ave S

S Norfolk St

0   200   400   600 yards

0   200   400   600 meters

5

30 rainier Beach and Kubota Garden: THE CITY'S LOWER EDGE

BOUNDARIES: Martin Luther King Jr. Way S., S. Henderson St., Seward Park Ave. S., and S. Norfolk St.
DISTANCE: 3½ miles
DIFFICULTY: Moderate (one uphill segment at the start)
PARKING: Free parking at Kubota Garden and at the Atlantic City Boat Ramp
PUBLIC TRANSIT: Link light rail stops at this walk's start; so do Metro routes #8, 9, 106, and 107.

One man's monument to the nurturing power of nature lies at the city's southeast corner. The Kubota Garden was part lifetime hobby, part professional showcase for its landscaper-builder. Now everyone's free to enjoy its 20 acres of hills, valleys, streams, ponds, and garden spaces designed with Japanese techniques and Northwest native plants. You'll get there via a walking path that's a little slice of electrified open space. This walk's back end returns you to the shores of Lake Washington, at a little jewel of a shoreline park.

● Start at the Rainier Beach light rail station, Martin Luther King Jr. Way S. and S. Henderson St. As with all the stations on the Central Link line, it's decorated with big, whimsical public art. The dominant piece here is Buster Simpson's *Parable,* a bowl of giant peaches cast in rusted iron, with old rail ties as stems. Across MLK Way there's a building shaped like a Hawaiian longhouse. It's the Vegetable Bin Polynesian Deli, selling both authentic island fare and convenience-store items.

● Walk east on Henderson for one block. Take a right turn onto the Chief Sealth Trail. It's a paved walking and biking path along a long, grassy open space, under the municipally-owned Seattle City Light's transmission towers. Since the city already had the land, turning it into a scenic walk was cheap. (The path's asphalt was reclaimed from the light rail line, which took out a couple lanes of street.) The whole trail runs 3½ miles; you wind southeast and a bit uphill on it for a half mile.

For a less scenic but flatter alternate route, continue east on Henderson beyond the intersection with the trail, then turn southeast onto Renton Ave. S.

- This segment of the trail empties into Marcus Ave. S., which takes a left turn into S. Roxbury St. Continue on the quiet, residential Roxbury to Renton Ave. S. Turn right onto Renton. Make another right at 55th Ave. S., which leads immediately to the entrance to Kubota Garden.

  Now a free city park, Kubota Garden was originally the private hobby and demonstration site for professional gardener Fujitaro Kubota (1879–1973). He and his family spent five decades developing the site, interrupted by the Japanese American internment during World War II. A portion of it is in the formal Japanese garden tradition. The rest was developed according to Kubota's own conception, drawing on an East-meets-West aesthetic. You can follow the map posted just inside the entrance, simply wander, or take a clockwise loop through the grounds' various sections (terrace, waterfall, mountainside, stroll garden, Japanese garden, and stone garden), returning to the entrance.

- Back at the garden gate, take a left back onto 55th, then take another left to backtrack on Renton Ave. for one block.

- Turn north on 54th Ave. S., making a right-left dogleg at S. Roxbury St. These are low-density blocks of homes that get fancier the closer they are to Lake

SIDE TRIP: SEWARD PARK

To make this walk longer, continue north on Seward Park Ave. S. beyond S. Henderson St. After 1¾ miles, turn east on S. Juneau St. and into Seward Park. The 300-acre nature park sits on its own peninsula. You can take a 3-mile walk around the lakefront, which includes a swimming beach, and follow inland trails through 120 acres of old-growth forest, teeming with plants and birds. Seward is also directly reachable on a #39 bus. More information is at the Friends of Seward Park website, sewardpark.org.

Washington. Continue on 54th to Rainier Ave. S. Turn east on Rainier for one long block, past affordable food spots of both indie and franchise varieties.

● Turn northwest onto Seward Park Ave. S. To your right, you pass a private marina and yacht club. Then you reach the public Atlantic City Boat Ramp, the southernmost of three adjacent city parks. There's some green space and some open shoreline just north of the dock, as the site segues into Beer Sheva Park (renamed after Seattle's Israeli sister city). If you've got the time, you can stroll a little farther north into Pritchard Island Beach Park. There's a beach there, but not an island. When the lake was lowered last century, a shallow slough between the mainland and a small private island became aboveground wetlands. Most of the Pritchard park is on this strip. The park also has a beach and a rental meeting hall.

● When you've finished visiting these parks, return to the intersection of Seward Park and Henderson, just north of the boat dock. Turn west on Henderson. To your right are Rainier Beach High School and the K–8 South Shore School. The latter campus includes Rainier Henderson Plaza, a handsome public square featuring a circular labyrinth path. (It's similar to the labyrinth at St. Paul's Episcopal Church in lower Queen Anne, Walk 8.) Free afternoon concerts are held here in the summer. The plaza adjoins the Rainier Beach Community Center, a large rental space for events of all types.

Continue west on Henderson, back to the Rainier Beach Station.

CONNECTING THE WALKS

This walk starts 2½ miles south of Walk 29's start.

POINTS OF INTEREST

Rainier Beach Station soundtransit.org, Martin Luther King Jr. Way S. and S. Henderson St.

Vegetable Bin Polynesian Deli 8816 Martin Luther King Jr. Way S., 206-725-0543

Kubota Garden kubota.org, 9817 55th Ave. S., 206-684-4584

Atlantic City Boat Ramp seattle.gov/parks/Boats/motorized.htm, 8702 Seward Park Ave. S., 206-684-7249

Beer Sheva Park seattle.gov/parks, 8650 55th Ave. S.

Rainier Beach High School rainierbeachhs.seattleschools.org, 8815 Seward Park Ave. S.

Rainier Beach Community Center and Playfield seattle.gov/parks/centers/rainierbeach.htm, 8825 Rainier Ave. S., 206-386-1925

route summary

1. Start on S. Henderson St., walking east from Martin Luther King Jr. Way S.
2. Turn onto the Chief Sealth Trail, winding southeast.
3. Turn east on S. Roxbury St.
4. Turn southeast on Renton Ave. S.
5. Turn south on 55th Ave. S. to Kubota Garden.
6. Take a clockwise loop through the garden, returning to the entrance.
7. Backtrack north on 55th and northwest on Renton.
8. Turn north on 54th Ave. S.
9. Dogleg right-left at S. Roxbury St. and back onto 54th.
10. Turn east on Rainier Ave. S.
11. Turn northwest on Seward Park Ave. S.
12. Turn west on Henderson, back to your start.

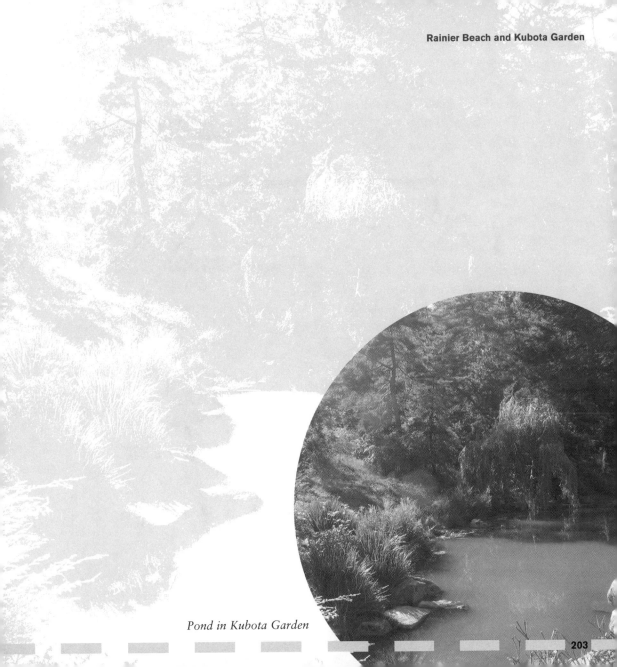

Pond in Kubota Garden

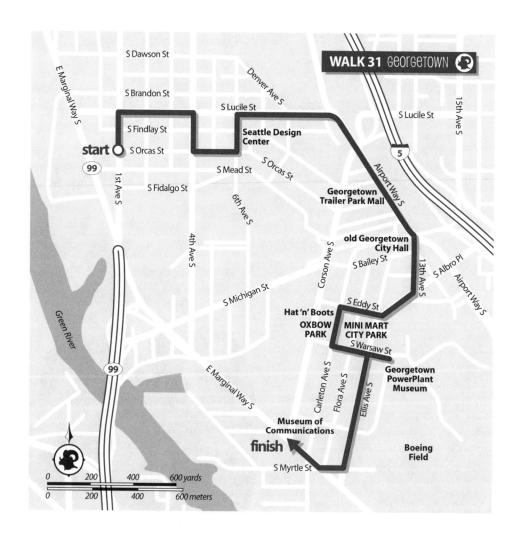

S Dawson St

S Brandon St

Denver Ave S

S Lucile St

S Lucile St

15th Ave S

E Marginal Way S

S Findlay St

Seattle Design Center

start ○ S Orcas St

99

1st Ave S

S Mead St

S Orcas St

5

Airport Way S

S Fidalgo St

6th Ave S

4th Ave S

Georgetown Trailer Park Mall

old Georgetown City Hall

S Bailey St

13th Ave S

S Albro Pl

Airport Way S

Corson Ave S

S Michigan St

Green River

99

S Eddy St

Hat 'n' Boots
OXBOW PARK

MINI MART CITY PARK

S Warsaw St

E Marginal Way S

Carleton Ave S

Flora Ave S

Ellis Ave S

Georgetown PowerPlant Museum

Museum of Communications

finish

Boeing Field

S Myrtle St

0   200   400   600 yards
0   200   400   600 meters

31 GeorGeTOWN: IN THe SHADOWS OF BOEING

BOUNDARIES: **1st Ave. S., Airport Way S., S. Lucile St., and 13th Ave. S.**
DISTANCE: **2½ miles**
DIFFICULTY: **Easy (all flat)**
PARKING: **Free street parking along S. Orcas St.**
PUBLIC TRANSIT: **Metro route #132 stops near this route's start.**

Georgetown, another of the former independent towns annexed into Seattle, is an urban island surrounded by industry, a freeway, two freight yards, and a cargo airport. In recent years, it has gone from neglected hamlet to arts mecca. This is partly because those decades of neglect had left a main street of rugged brick and metal-clad post-frontier storefronts, across from the quarter-mile long edifice of a pre-Prohibition brewing plant. These spaces nurtured what *Seattle Weekly* writer Laura Cassidy called a style of "post-squat, industrial bohemian chic." Georgetown's residential streets have their own charm, with many ornate Victorian and Edwardian home styles you won't find in most of Seattle. You'll also see a genuine piece of reclaimed 1950s roadside kitsch, and a couple of new hangouts styled as homages to roadside kitsch.

● Start on the east side of 1st Ave. S., walking north from S. Orcas St. You soon spot the retro-roadhouse facade of Slim's Last Chance Chili Shack. The kitsch-nostalgia diner, saloon, and music spot is just as whimsical inside. A similar vibe carries on next door at Iron Pig BBQ.

● Turn east on S. Lucile St. at the fab '50s neon of the La Hacienda Motel, one of many that once flourished along and near US 99 in the pre-interstate era. Approaching 4th Ave. S., you pass a garden statuary lot (always fun to look at). Across 4th, the Vac Shop displays a variety of classic vacuums out front, along with at least one '50s sci-fi robot and a sign promoting FREE BIBLES INSIDE.

● Turn south on 4th for two blocks. At 4th and Orcas, the Marco Polo is a comfy neighborhood sports bar with exceptional fried chicken.

● Turn back onto Orcas, heading east. To your left, the Tiger Lounge is a cute little bungalow all repainted in retro-mod colors. It offers bistro lunches by day, hopping dance music by night. The much, much bigger building to your right is the Seattle Design Center, filled with home-furnishings showrooms. It's normally open only to interior designers and contractors, but some tenants have occasional sample sales. You can also get a guided tour from a matchmaker who'll connect you to a home-design pro.

- Turn north on 6th Ave. S. and continue for two blocks back to Lucile. Walk east for four blocks on Lucile, past loading docks and low-rise offices, toward Airport Way S., Georgetown's main drag.

- Turn southeast onto the right side of Airport Way. It runs for nearly a half mile of recent, older, and really old low-rise storefronts and ex-hotels. Some look like Old West movie sets. Some look like standard neighborhood-retail buildings. Some are more (and more authentically) restored than others. All this variety simply adds to the strip's funky charm. The first arty joints you see are Great Stuff Vintage Furnishings and Georgetown Liquor Co. (a bar and veggie restaurant). A little farther down, Stellar Pizza serves up cool mod design and vintage pinball games along with its food and drinks. Just west of Airport on Corson Ave. S., the Corson Building is an intimate ultra-foodie restaurant, serving local organic ingredients in a 1910 Spanish-eclectic building behind a rose-covered iron fence.

- Cross Corson, under a freeway on-ramp, to continue down Airport Way. To your left, you soon see the sprawling brick edifices of Rainier Brewing's pre-Prohibition plant. Its tenants include several art studios, open on second Saturday art walks. (Rainier's post-Repeal production was at an equally historic site, two miles north of here.) To your right, the funky, artsy storefronts continue with the Georgetown Ballroom, Two Tartes Bakery, the old-timey restaurants and bars Calamity Jane's and Jules Maes, Full Throttle Bottles (a beer-wine store with a music and meeting space in back), and the Georgetown Trailer Park Mall (art, antiques, and vintage clothes sold in vintage camping trailers).

South of S. Vale St., just beyond the Big Peoples Scooter lot (headquarters of the Vespa revival), the Horton Building is ground zero of the Georgetown arts scene. In this full-block former hotel are the 9 Lb. Hammer bar, the Smarty Pants soup and

SIDE TRIP: MUSEUM OF FLIGHT

Situated at Boeing Field's southwest end, the Museum of Flight celebrates Seattle's heritage as the world capital of commercial aircraft and a major center for aviation in general. It incorporates William Boeing's original "Red Barn" factory, plus permanent and rotating displays covering a century of human flight. The museum's own collection includes more than 150 historic aircraft, spacecraft, and associated artifacts.

sandwich restaurant, the All City Coffee espresso joint, Georgetown Records (vintage vinyl kings), the Fantagraphics Bookstore and Gallery (retail outlet for the leading graphic novel publishers in the United States), a recording studio, and artist live and work spaces. On the southern wall is artist Kathryn Rathke's neon sign depicting Georgetown landmarks beneath the face of a lady shushing at a loud airplane approaching Boeing Field.

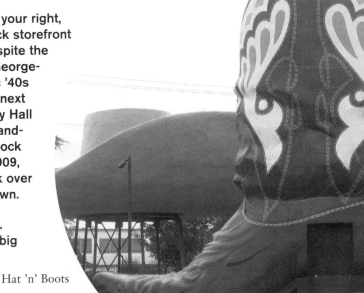

- Turn south on 13th Ave. S. To your right, the Miller Building, a 1929 brick storefront block, still looks gorgeous despite the recent loss of the venerable Georgetown Pharmacy and its classic '40s neon sign. To your left on the next block, the old Georgetown City Hall is a handsome two-story red-and-white structure with a small clock tower on top. It was built in 1909, just a year before Seattle took over the previously independent town.

- Turn southwest on S. Albro Pl. To your left in the distance, a big

Hat 'n' Boots

checkerboard wall marks the visual approach for aircraft approaching King County Airport-Boeing Field. The region's first major airfield, it's now used mostly for cargo, charters, and general aviation. Farther along Albro, you see and smell floral goodies at Rosso Nursery, a spot of organic beauty next to the aircraft hangars.

● Turn west on S. Eddy St. for two blocks; then turn south on Carleton Ave. S. To your right halfway down the block, a former vacant lot is now Oxbow Park. The pocket park is named for a bend in the Duwamish River, that was taken out when the river was redredged to be more barge-friendly. The park is home to the *Hat 'n' Boots*. This giant cowboy hat, man's boot, and woman's boot were originally the office and rest-rooms of a '50s gas station on nearby East Marginal Way S. The city moved the road-side attractions, which volunteers then restored.

Across Carleton, the turreted Victorian Georgetown Castle is the location of frequent alleged ghost sightings. The Travel Channel called it one of the most terrifying places in America. You can see it on guided tours every Halloween season.

● Turn east on S. Warsaw St. At the northwest corner of Warsaw and Ellis Ave. S., Mini Mart City Park is a 1930s gas station taken over by conceptual artists John Sutton, Ben Beres, and Zac Culler. They plan to turn it into a landscaped public green space, once the soil has been decontaminated or replaced.

Continue one more block on Warsaw toward the Georgetown Steam Plant, a 1906 oil- and coal-powered electric generating station. Most of its equipment is still installed and kept in good shape by a volunteer group, the Georgetown PowerPlant Museum. The building also hosts a model-train club, the Puget Sound Garden Railway Society. The two groups hold open houses the second Saturday of each month. Most of the rest of the time, you have to view the handsome structure (one of the first reinforced-concrete buildings on the Pacific Coast) from behind a fence.

● Return to Warsaw and Ellis. Turn left (south) on Ellis. To your right, you see working-class homes in various degrees of fanciness and upkeep. To your left, warehouses and truck lots. Behind that, the west side of Boeing Field.

● Turn west on S. Myrtle St. for two blocks; then turn northwest on the right side of East Marginal for two more blocks. You pass the Airlane, an old flophouse-style hotel still in use, and the forlorn sign of the closed Chief Seattle Motel. The Museum of Communications, a volunteer-curated collection of analog-era telephone gear, is in an old Bell System switching center at East Marginal and Corson Ave. S. It's open Tuesdays or by appointment.

● From here you can take a #124 bus back to 4th and Orcas. Or you can walk 2 miles southeast on East Marginal, or take a southbound #124, to the Museum of Flight at Boeing Field's southern end.

CONNECTING THE WALKS

This walk starts 1¼ miles south of Walk 12.

POINTS OF INTEREST

Slim's Last Chance Chili Shack slimslastchance.com, 5506 1st Ave. S., 206-762-7900

Seattle Design Center seattledesigncenter.com, 5701 6th Ave. S., 800-497-7997

Georgetown Trailer Park Mall georgetowntrailerpark.com, 947 Doris St.

Georgetown Records and Fantagraphics Books georgetownrecords.net and fantagraphics.com, 1201 S. Vale St., 206-762-5638

Georgetown PowerPlant Museum nps.gov/history/nr/travel/seattle/s35.htm, 6605 13th Ave. S., 206-763-2542

Oxbow Park seattle.gov/parks, 6425 Carleton Ave. S

Georgetown Castle georgetownhistory.com, 6420 Carleton Ave. S

Mini Mart City Park minimartcitypark.com, 6525 Ellis Ave. S., 206-722-2116

Museum of Communications museumofcommunications.org, 7000 East Marginal Way S., 206-767-3012

Museum of Flight museumofflight.org, 9409 E. Marginal Way, 206-764-5700

route summary

1. Start on 1st Ave. S., walking north from S. Orcas St.
2. Turn east on S. Lucile St.
3. Turn south on 4th Ave. S.
4. Turn east back onto Orcas.
5. Turn north on 6th Ave. S.
6. Turn east back onto Lucile.
7. Turn southeast on Airport Way S.
8. Turn south on 13th Ave. S.
9. Turn southwest on S. Albro Pl.
10. Turn west on S. Eddy St.
11. Turn south on Carleton Ave. S.
12. Turn east on S. Warsaw St. for three blocks, then backtrack one block.
13. Turn south on Ellis Ave. S.
14. Turn west on S. Myrtle St.
15. Turn northwest on East Marginal Way S., to Corson Ave. S.

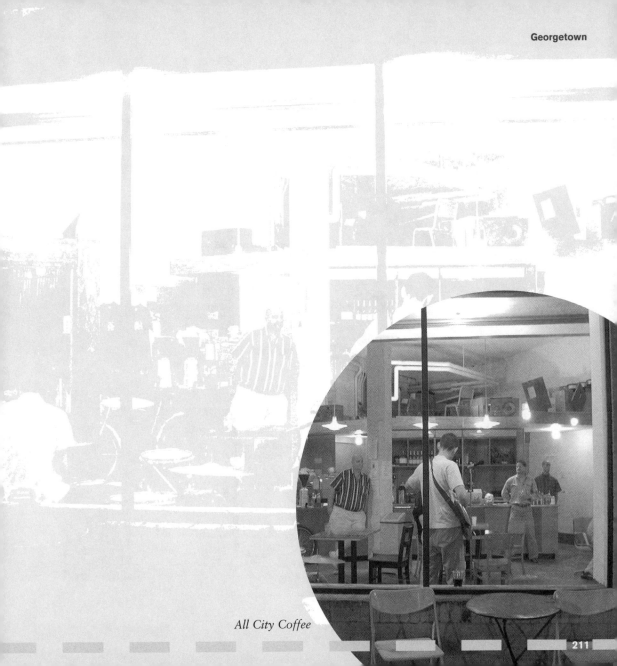

All City Coffee

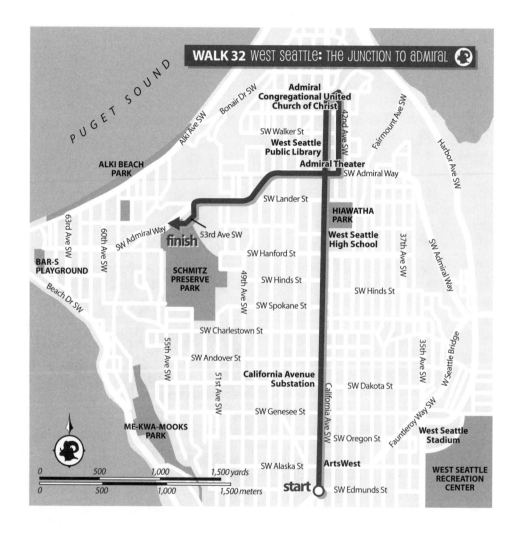

PUGET SOUND

Admiral Congregational United Church of Christ

SW Walker St

West Seattle Public Library

Admiral Theater

SW Admiral Way

SW Lander St

ALKI BEACH PARK

Alki Ave SW

Bonair Dr SW

42nd Ave SW

Fairmount Ave SW

Harbor Ave SW

HIAWATHA PARK

West Seattle High School

37th Ave SW

SW Admiral Way

SW Admiral Way

53rd Ave SW

finish

63rd Ave SW

60th Ave SW

BAR-S PLAYGROUND

Beach Dr SW

SCHMITZ PRESERVE PARK

49th Ave SW

SW Hanford St

SW Hinds St

SW Hinds St

SW Spokane St

SW Charlestown St

55th Ave SW

SW Andover St

51st Ave SW

California Avenue Substation

California Ave SW

SW Dakota St

35th Ave SW

W Seattle Bridge

SW Genesee St

ME-KWA-MOOKS PARK

SW Oregon St

Fauntleroy Way SW

West Seattle Stadium

SW Alaska St

ArtsWest

start

SW Edmunds St

WEST SEATTLE RECREATION CENTER

| 0 | 500 | 1,000 | 1,500 yards |
| 0 | 500 | 1,000 | 1,500 meters |

32 WeST SeaTTLe: THe JUNCTION TO aDMIRaL: a CITY WITHIN THe CITY

BOUNDARIES: **SW Edmunds St., 42nd Ave. SW, SW Admiral Way, and SW Stevens St.**
DISTANCE: **3½ miles**
DIFFICULTY: **Moderate (two brief uphill segments toward the end)**
PARKING: **Free street parking and pay lots**
PUBLIC TRANSIT: **Metro routes #22, 54, 55, 57, and 128 stop near this route's start.**

West Seattle lies on a separate peninsula from the rest of the city, and sometimes seems like a separate world. Our last four walks traverse different parts of it, beginning with its commercial and transit hub. The Junction was named after the streetcar lines that intersected it, creating the obvious site for West Seattle's business district. Like many of the neighborhood retail strips you've seen in this book, it's now abloom with cool independent stores, galleries, restaurants, and bars. Your trek continues past a classic high school building and a nautical-themed movie theater. It ends at one of the city's last patches of never-logged forest land.

● Start on California Ave. SW, walking north from SW Edmunds St. This is the start of the Junction, West Seattle's principal shopping district. This first long block comprises some standard American one- and two-story main street storefronts. Many offer traditional main-street wares—furniture, bedding, pet supplies, and prescriptions. Others are a little more uncommon, such as Bakery Nouveau (butter croissants to die for), Husky Deli (homestyle ice cream to kill for), ArtsWest (a theater and art gallery), and Rubato Records (rare vinyl and music memorabilia).

The next intersection is California and SW Alaska St. The Junction got its name from the streetcar lines that used to cross here. It's still a major bus transfer point. To your left just beyond Alaska, Easy Street Records and Cafe is a full-service music outlet plus a full-service diner. As one of the store's ad slogans explains: "Because downloads don't come with fries." Next door on Alaska, the Twilight Artist Collective (no relation to the vampire novels set in Washington but written in Arizona) sells both traditional artworks and designer products from local artists (scarves, T-shirts, purses, magnets, tiles, and more).

As you resume your northbound trek on California, you pass three more long blocks of storefronts. They include antique shops, a yoga studio, used-book stores, jewelers, a model-train shop, a rubber-stamp shop, coffeehouses, teahouses, snack shops, and lounge restaurants. Two favorites among the latter include the funky-but-chic West 5 and the exquisitely posh Jak's Grill. There are also handsome low-rise churches, West Seattle Baptist and Olympic Lutheran.

To your left just north of SW Dakota St., the former California Avenue Substation is a '30s neo-classical brick box with terra-cotta ornamentation. It's also a remnant of the era (1901–1951) when Seattle had two competing electric companies, the city-owned City Light and the private Seattle Electric (later renamed Puget Power, still operating in the suburbs as Puget Sound Energy). North of that, and for the next several blocks, California becomes a quiet tree-lined arterial, mostly occupied by midcentury homes and apartments. One commercial interruption is the Charlestown Street Cafe, specializing in Charlestown chowder.

To your left near California and SW Hinds St., a German-style pub and two indie pizza places mark the start of the Admiral district. To your right a little farther north lie the recently enlarged West Seattle High School and the adjacent Hiawatha Playfield. The school's original facade, built in 1917, bears a number of ancient symbols of varying origins, from pentacles and Greek crosses to ram's-head gargoyles.

● Wiseman's Appliance and TV, a throwback to the days of small neighborhood appliance stores (only with all new merchandise), stands just south of California and SW Admiral Way, the Admiral district's main intersection. Just north of it, on your left, the nautical-themed Admiral Theater still bears much of its '40s Art Moderne charm, despite an unfortunate 1973 "upgrade" that removed or covered up a lot of its cool decor. Three blocks farther north, as the street segues back into residential use, Admiral Congregational Church is an angular, monochromatic monument of early '60s Modernism tucked behind a pocket park.

● Turn northeast on Ferry Ave. SW for one block; then immediately turn south on 42nd Ave. SW for four blocks. This stretch starts in a quiet residential zone with big trees and shrubbery and transitions at the West Seattle Public Library on SW College St. This elegant brick structure was built in 1910 with an Andrew Carnegie grant. Just south of it is a Metropolitan Market upscale grocery, across from a bubble-era condo and retail behemoth.

- Turn west on SW Admiral Way, back toward the intersection with California. To your right, just beyond the Shipwreck Tavern, is the Heartland Cafe and Benbow Room. From 1950 to 2002 it was the Admiral Benbow Inn, a legendary comfort-food eatery and hangout bar. Its new owners faithfully restored the bar's Spanish-galleon theme, with fake sunlight streaming through stained-glass aft windows. Just west of California, Atomic Boys combines nostalgic candy and junk food with funky retro toys, games, and novelties.

- Continue on Admiral. It becomes a wide residential arterial, wending southwest and downhill, then west again. In the distance you can see a peep of the waters off of Alki Point (Walk 33).

- Turn south onto 53rd Ave. SW, initially a bit uphill. Your perseverance with this late incline will prove worth it once 53rd bends west into SW Stevens St., offering a magnificent view of Puget Sound and (on a good day) the Olympic Mountains.

Just before Stevens reunites with Admiral, you're at the north entrance to Schmitz Preserve Park. These 53 acres comprise some of the last old-growth woods left within the Seattle city limits. This land has been pretty much left in the state it was in when it was donated to the city, in tracts between 1908 and 1912. What work has been done on it has been to restore more of its original appearance, by taking out an interior parking lot and "daylighting" a creek that had been hidden in underground drainpipes.

- From here you can wander through Schmitz. Or you can return to Admiral Way and take a #56 bus back to California, then transfer to a #51, 55, or 128 bus back to the Junction.

CONNECTING THE WALKS

This walk connects easily with two other walks. It starts three-quarters of a mile north of Walk 35's start. At Ferry Ave. SW you're a half mile southwest of Walk 33.

POINTS OF INTEREST

Husky Deli huskydeli.com, 4721 California Ave. SW, 206-937-2810

ArtsWest artswest.org, 4711 California Ave. SW, 206-938-0963

Easy Street Records and Cafe easystreetonline.com, 4559 California Ave. SW, 206-938-3279

Charlestown Street Cafe charlestownchowder.com, 3800 California Ave. SW, 206-937-3800

West Seattle High School westseattlehs.seattleschools.org, 3000 California Ave. SW

Admiral Theater farawayentertainment.com/admiral.html, 2343 California Ave. SW, 206-938-0360

Admiral Congregational United Church of Christ admiralchurch.org, 4320 SW Hill St., 206-932-2928

Heartland Cafe and Benbow Room heartlandcafeseattle.com, 4210 SW Admiral Way, 206-922-3313

Atomic Boys atomicboysseattle.com, 4311 SW Admiral Way, 206-938-3255

Schmitz Preserve Park seattle.gov/parks, 5551 SW Admiral Way

route summary

1. Start on California Ave. SW, walking north from SW Edmunds St.
2. Continue on California past the Junction and Admiral business districts.
3. Turn northeast on Ferry Ave. SW.
4. Turn south on 42nd Ave. SW.
5. Turn west on SW Admiral Way S., past California and wending southwest.
6. Turn south on 53rd Ave. SW, which bends west into SW Stevens St. at the entrance to Schmitz Preserve Park.

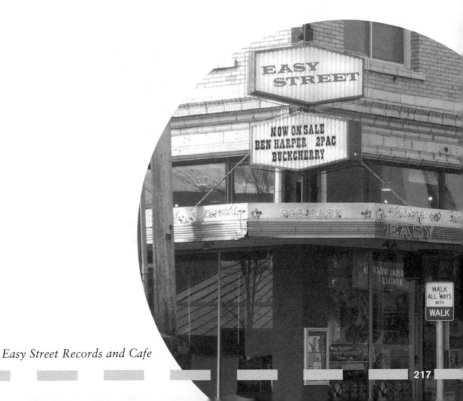

Easy Street Records and Cafe

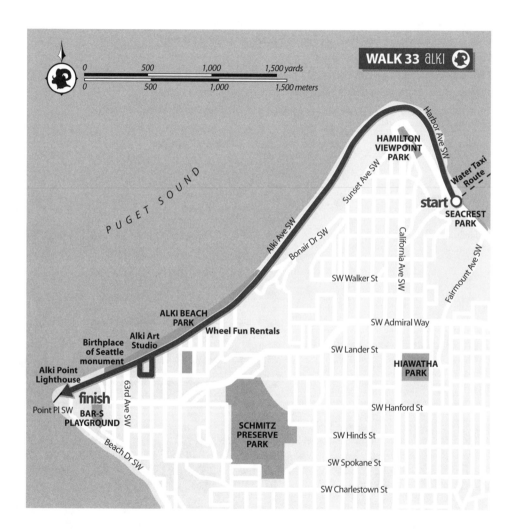

0   500   1,000   1,500 yards
0   500   1,000   1,500 meters

PUGET SOUND

Harbor Ave SW

HAMILTON
VIEWPOINT
PARK

Sunset Ave SW

Water Taxi
Route

start ○
SEACREST
PARK

Alki Ave SW

Bonair Dr SW

California Ave SW

Fairmount Ave SW

SW Walker St

SW Admiral Way

ALKI BEACH
PARK

Wheel Fun Rentals

Alki Art
Studio

SW Lander St

HIAWATHA
PARK

Birthplace
of Seattle
monument

Alki Point
Lighthouse

finish

63rd Ave SW

SW Hanford St

Point Pl SW

BAR-S
PLAYGROUND

SCHMITZ
PRESERVE
PARK

SW Hinds St

Beach Dr SW

SW Spokane St

SW Charlestown St

33 ALKI: WHERE SEATTLE (REALLY) STARTED

BOUNDARIES: **Harbor Ave. SW, California Way SW, and the foot of Alki Ave. SW**
DISTANCE: **3¼ miles**
DIFFICULTY: **Easy (all flat, mostly on pedestrian-bicycle paths)**
PARKING: **Free but scarce street parking near Seacrest Park**
PUBLIC TRANSIT: **King County Water Taxi from the downtown waterfront or Metro routes #37 and 56**

On a miserable November day in 1851, 10 adults and 12 children landed in a schooner on a windswept beach to meet David Denny, who'd arrived before to scout possible settlement sites. They named their dreary outpost "New York-Alki" ("New York by-and-by" in Chinook Jargon). The following spring, the settlers mostly moved east to today's Pioneer Square. Alki later blossomed into a residential and recreational neighborhood. The city preserved several miles of the Puget Sound shore for public use. Depending on the season, you could find yourself walking here among hundreds of inline skaters, bicyclists, and parents pushing baby strollers, or among just a few diehard joggers. The walk leads you to Alki Beach, a highly popular site for sea gazing and socializing (and, during the peak years of the hot-rod culture, for car cruising).

● **Start at Seacrest Park, perhaps by taking the King County Water Taxi from Pier 50 downtown. If you drive to Seacrest, be warned that street parking is often filled by Water Taxi commuters. Seacrest's best-known asset is a spectacular view of the downtown skyline, seen in such films as** The Fabulous Baker Boys. **The park also offers a public fishing pier, a boat launch, and a fish-and-chips stand.**

● **Turn northwest onto Harbor Ave. SW. If you like, you can partake at the Alki Tavern (an ungentrified dive bar) a little up the road.**

● **Continue as this glorious promenade bends southwest at Duwamish Head, becoming Alki Ave. SW. This is where you'll find the city's monument to Luna Park, an amusement pier that operated from 1912 until an arsonist torched it in 1933. Old photos depict it as a gloriously tacky, Edwardian pleasure spot. As you walk farther, you find more city-installed monuments to Alki's past and to local sea creatures and plants.**

Keep going a leisurely 2 miles on the street's west side, which faces an open, public shore. You may be accompanied by many other walkers, strollers, bicyclists, and roller-skaters. (Icons on the wide sidewalk tell you which lane to stay in to avoid a bicycle and pedestrian pile-up.)

Note two types of residential structures along the street's east side, hulking condominiums and quaint little cottages. While the cottages look more rustic and cozy, they were originally just as "upscale" as the condos—most were built as summer homes for the well-to-do. This stretch is known to some locals as the "pipeline," after an old street runoff pipe buried in rock. It's alternately called the "junkyard," after decades-old household debris that appears at low tide.

The shorefront park widens into a broad beach. The bluff behind the condos and cottages gives way to a gentler slope. Older apartment buildings appear on the landward side of the street, as does the start of the Alki business district. Among the first businesses you see is Wheel Fun Rentals, a bicycle rental franchise.

Shortly beyond that is the homey Pepperdock Restaurant, a good place for fish-and-chips and burgers. More dining options await down the street, at a full range of price points. The Alki business strip has become a restaurant row, to the exclusion of most other business types (its only supermarket closed in 2002). Its oldest occupant is Spud Fish & Chips, first opened in 1935.

Back on the beach is Alki Park's only building, the historic Alki Bathhouse. It's been remodeled to contain a community meeting hall and public art studios.

● Farther down the beach is a miniature Statue of Liberty on a lighthouse-shaped pedestal, a 2008 replacement for a statue donated by the Boy Scouts in 1952 (it became an instant gathering spot for folks depositing flowers and mementos after 9/11). You can see the previous copy on display at the Log House Museum, mentioned later in this walk.

● Turn back, cross Alki Ave. at 61st Ave. SW, and walk east a half block to the Alki Homestead Restaurant, built in 1903 as the Fir Lodge. The restaurant's been closed since a 2009 fire, but you can still admire its bulky log-cabin structure and its stoic vertical neon sign.

- Farther down on 61st, past SW Stevens St., you find the Log House Museum. It was originally the carriage house for the building now known as the Alki Homestead. It houses neighborhood mementos and exhibits.

- Return to Alki Ave. and 61st. Cross the street to return to Alki Beach Park, then continue southwest until you reach the *Birthplace of Seattle,* a white obelisk marking the first white settlement in present-day Seattle on November 13, 1851. It was revised in 2001 to include the female settlers' first names, and to recognize the Native peoples who were already here. Its base includes a fragment of Plymouth Rock, installed in 1926.

- Recross Alki Ave. at 64th Ave. SW. Tucked inconspicuously on this quiet residential street you'll find Seattle's oldest existing house at 3045 64th. It's a modest brown structure with cedar trim, built circa 1858 for city cofounder Dr. David S. "Doc" May-nard (a legendary character given more to gregariousness and liquor than to monu-mental architecture). If it doesn't look "historic," that's because it's been expanded and facelifted several times.

- Backtracking to Alki Ave. lets you check out some whimsical apartment structures, includ-ing one vaguely shaped like a series of ship's sails. Too bad the recent condo-building craze has included little or none of this architectural creativity.

- Another half mile down Alki Ave., past the end of the public beach, is the stately white Alki Point Lighthouse. Built in 1913, it's open for tours on weekend summer afternoons. The rest of the time, you might skip this segment of the walk; there's not even a good spot to look at the lighthouse from the street.

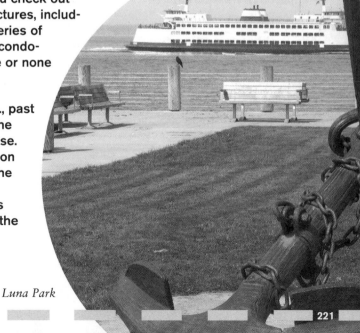

Luna Park

● Backtrack to Alki Drive and 61st. From here, you can take a free shuttle bus back to the Water Taxi, or take a #37 or 56 bus to the Admiral district (Walk 32) and downtown.

CONNECTING THE WALKS

This walk connects easily with five other walks. The Water Taxi brings you to the central Waterfront (Walk 7), which is also near the Pike Place Market (Walk 4), the downtown retail core (Walks 2 and 3), and Pioneer Square (Walk 1).

POINTS OF INTEREST

King County Water Taxi, Pier 50 kingcountyferries.org, Alaskan Way and Yesler Way, 206-684-1511

Seacrest Park seattle.gov/parks, 1660 Harbor Ave. SW

Alki Beach Park seattle.gov/parks, 1702 Alki Ave. SW

Pepperdock Restaurant 2618 Alki Ave. SW, 206-935-1000

Spud Fish & Chips spudfishandchips.com, 2666 Alki Ave. SW, 206-938-0606

Alki Bathhouse and Art Studios seattle.gov/parks/arts/alkiart.htm, 2701 Alki Ave. SW, 206-684-7430

Alki Homestead Restaurant 2717 61st Ave. SW

Log House Museum loghousemuseum.info, 3003 61st Ave. SW, 206-938-5293

Alki Point Lighthouse uscg.mil/history/weblighthouses/LHWA.asp, 3201 Alki Ave. SW, 206-841-3519

route summary

1. Start at Seacrest Park, perhaps by taking the King County Water Taxi from Pier 55 downtown.
2. Turn northwest onto Harbor Ave. SW, which becomes Alki Ave. SW.
3. Turn east on 61st Ave. SW.
4. Turn west on SW Stevens St.
5. Turn north on 62nd Ave. SW.
6. Return to Alki; walk southwest to the *Birthplace of Seattle* monument.
7. Turn east on 64th Ave. SW a half block to the Doc Maynard house. Backtrack to Alki.
8. Resume going southwest on Alki Ave. to the Alki Point Lighthouse.
9. Return to Alki Ave. and 61st.

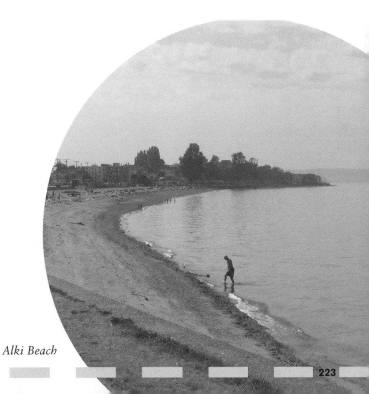

Alki Beach

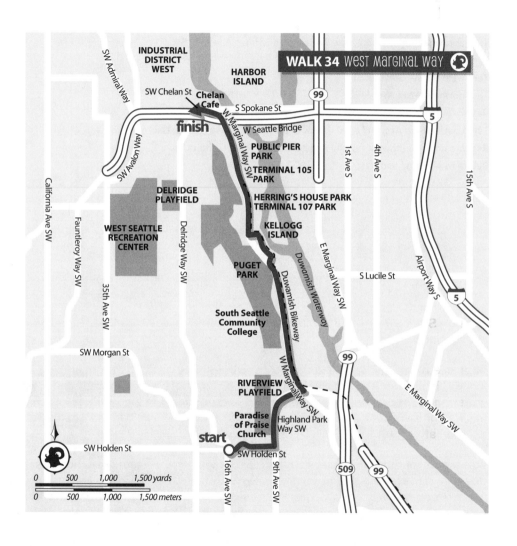

SW Admiral Way

INDUSTRIAL
DISTRICT
WEST

HARBOR
ISLAND

SW Chelan St

Chelan
Cafe

S Spokane St

99

5

finish

W Marginal Way SW

W Seattle Bridge

SW Avalon Way

California Ave SW

Fauntleroy Way SW

35th Ave SW

DELRIDGE
PLAYFIELD

Delridge Way SW

WEST SEATTLE
RECREATION
CENTER

PUBLIC PIER
PARK

TERMINAL 105
PARK

HERRING'S HOUSE PARK
TERMINAL 107 PARK

KELLOGG
ISLAND

PUGET
PARK

Duwamish Waterway

Duwamish Bikeway

South Seattle
Community
College

1st Ave S

4th Ave S

15th Ave S

E Marginal Way SW

S Lucile St

Airport Way S

5

SW Morgan St

RIVERVIEW
PLAYFIELD

99

Paradise
of Praise
Church

Highland Park
Way SW

W Marginal Way SW

E Marginal Way SW

start

SW Holden St

16th Ave SW

SW Holden St

9th Ave SW

509

99

0   500   1,000   1,500 yards
0   500   1,000   1,500 meters

34 WeST MarGiNaL WaY: WHere NaTure MeeTS carGo

BOUNDARIES: 16th Ave. SW, SW Holden St., W. Marginal Way SW, and SW Chelan St.
DISTANCE: 4 miles
DIFFICULTY: Moderate (almost all flat or downhill)
PARKING: Free street parking
PUBLIC TRANSIT: Metro routes #125 and 128 stop near this route's start.

"The Real West Marginal Way," to quote the title of the late local poet Richard Hugo's autobiography, is a place where shipping and heavy industry exist side by side with pieces of restored natural settings along the Duwamish River. The river itself, the original birthplace of Boeing airplanes and Kenworth trucks, was redredged and rerouted decades ago, to provide a deeper and straighter passage for ocean-bound freighters. In recent years, a walking and biking path has been added along West Marginal, along with a series of small parks that recreate pieces of the original Duwamish environment. Your walk starts with a downhill hike through a "greenbelt," one of Seattle's stretches of protected woodlands.

● Start on SW Holden Street, walking east from 16th Ave. SW in West Seattle's deep residential heartland.

● After one block, Holden curves northeast, then southeast. The most striking building along this stretch is the Paradise of Praise Church. It's an asymmetrical, woodframe storefront church that looks older than it is (built only in 1995). Otherwise, this six-block segment mostly has modest homes and simple '60s-era apartments, interspersed after 12th Ave. SW with rows of bubble-era townhomes.

● Turn north on the right side of Highland Park Way SW. This street bends east and downhill through the West Duwamish Greenbelt, a huge canopy of second-growth forest along the West Seattle peninsula's eastern bluff, preserved partly to help prevent erosion. You'll think you're on a gently curving country road, at least until the semis career by. Fortunately, you've got a separate walking and biking lane to the east of the road. To your left approaching the bottom of the hill, a sign invites you onto a network of trails through the greenbelt.

● This rural vibe ends promptly once you reach the bottom of the hill. The Duwamish River's working waterfront comes into view, along with West Marginal Way SW. Cross at the light to the northeast corner of this intersection.

● From there head north on the Duwamish Bikeway paralleling West Marginal's east side. To your left, the Duwamish Greenbelt continues, occasionally interrupted by warehouses and metalwork plants. (This part of the greenbelt has especially scenic fall foliage.) To your right, you see Portside Coffee, an espresso stand shaped like the bow of a steel merchant ship.

North of Portside is a huge freight yard, with cargo containers stacked up like huge Lego constructions. North of that are cement and asphalt plants that were quite busy during the construction boom years, but are slightly less so nowadays. They're still magnificent structures, highlighted by big gray cylindrical towers huddled together in clumps.

● Just north of these plants, the bikeway takes a dogleg detour away from West Marginal and toward Terminal 107 Park. It's one of several waterfront park

SIDE TRIP: SOUTH SEATTLE COMMUNITY COLLEGE

South Seattle Community College's north side has a fastidiously landscaped 6-acre arboretum. Created in 1978, it serves both as an elegant walking and picnicking spot and as a living laboratory for the school's landscape-horticulture program. It also includes a student-run garden store.

Next to the arboretum is the Seattle Chinese Garden. This 4.5-acre hilltop site is still under construction as this book goes to press. But it already offers a magnificent outdoor pavilion plus tremendous views of the Duwamish Greenbelt bluff and the Duwamish Waterway. The college itself has a renowned culinary arts department. It operates three on-campus restaurants (from cafeteria-style to formal dining) and a pastry shop.

spaces recently added along the Duwamish. The Port of Seattle built them under a city law requiring the port to add public space whenever it remodels a shipping facility. This one has nearly a half mile of public shoreline, put back into a more-or-less natural state with the help of the nonprofit People for Puget Sound. It has views of Kellogg Island, a tiny islet that's also been deindustrialized. It has eagles, ospreys, and migrating salmon. (Signs warn against eating fish caught here.)

- Continue north as the port-owned Terminal 107 Park segues seamlessly into the city-owned Herring's House Park. The name is a translation of the original Duwamish tribal name for this spot. Archaeologists believe the area around this riverbank has been inhabited by humans for more than 1,400 years. (So much for the notion of pre-white Seattle as barren wilderness.) The city's section of the park includes a natural intertidal basin at the shoreline, along with areas of marsh, meadow, forest, and a narrow beach. It also features a five-eighths-scale model of a 1920s fishing boat. Its creator, artist Donald Fels, modeled it after boats that were made at shops that once stood at this site.

- Return from the park to the bikeway, walking north. To your left, you soon spot the Duwamish Longhouse and Cultural Center. The Duwamish tribal headquarters is the first new tribal longhouse built in Seattle in more than 140 years. It's home to art exhibits, performances, and community events.

- The bikeway ends just beyond here. Turn onto West Marginal. The street bends northwest here, past warehouses, bus lots, a kitchen-supply showroom, and a metals-products distributor with the cute name "Metal Shorts."

- Just north of the intersection of West Marginal and SW Dakota St., there's a narrow paved pathway behind an open gate to your right. It's the road to Terminal 105 Park, another Port of Seattle public space project. Along with 220 feet of restored shoreline, it's got a fishing pier, a launch for nonmotorized boats, a restored mudflat for fish to feed, public restrooms, and a picnic area with great views of the river and Mt. Rainier.

- Cross to West Marginal's left side, the only side where there's now a sidewalk. Resume walking northwest. To your right there's another big cement plant and a diving and salvage company. To your left, a narrow, two-story, brick-front office building with arched windows is an island of dignified vintage architecture in these more rough-hewn environs. Behind it are 16th and 17th avenues, short residential streets with pre-1940 rooming houses and shotgun houses.

● Just before you walk beneath the tall **West Seattle Bridge**, the old Riverside Mill now houses a motor-freight yard; a sign commemorates the property's lumber-making past. Continue on West Marginal as it bends west, becoming Chelan Ave. SW at the Chelan Cafe (Walk 12).

● To get back to your start, cross to Chelan and SW Spokane St. and catch a #125 bus. If you've got the time and energy, consider a stopover along the #125 route at South Seattle Community College (see sidebar, page 226).

CONNECTING THE WALKS

This walk connects easily to two other walks. It ends at the same place as Walk 12. At West Marginal and Highland Park Way you're 1¼ miles from Walk 31, across the 1st Avenue S. bridge.

POINTS OF INTEREST

Paradise of Praise Church paradiseofpraise.org, 1316 SW Holden St., 206-764-1053

West Duwamish Greenbelt and Puget Park seattle.gov/parks, Highland Park Way SW and West Marginal Way SW

Portside Coffee 6720 West Marginal Way SW

Terminal 107 Park portseattle.org, 4700 West Marginal Way SW

Duwamish Longhouse and Cultural Center duwamishtribe.org, 4705 West Marginal Way SW, 206-431-1582

Terminal 105 Park portseattle.org, 4260 West Marginal Way SW

Chelan Cafe 3527 Chelan Ave. SW, 206-932-7383

South Seattle Community College southseattle.edu, 6000 16th Ave. SW, 206-764-5300

route summary

1. Start on SW Holden Street, walking east from 16th Ave. SW.

2. Turn north on Highland Park Way SW, which bends east and downhill.

3. Cross West Marginal Way SW. Turn north on the Duwamish Bikeway paralleling West Marginal's east side.

4. At the bikeway's northern end, turn onto West Marginal, continuing as the street bends northwest.

5. Continue on West Marginal as it bends west, to Chelan Ave. SW.

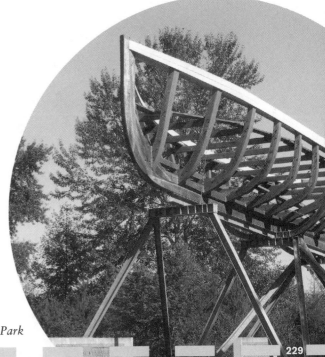

Scale model of a fishing boat in Herring's House Park

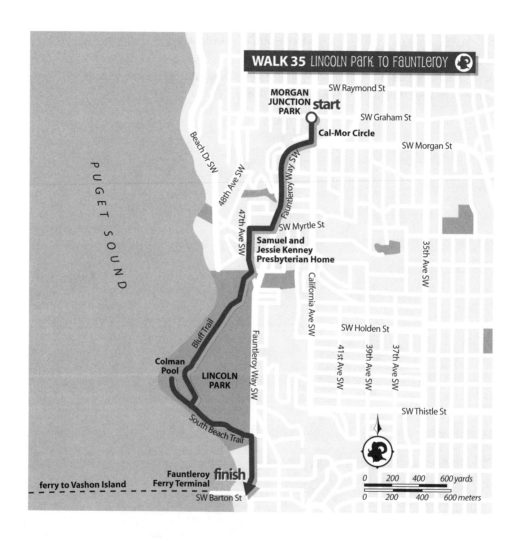

SW Raymond St

MORGAN JUNCTION PARK **start**

SW Graham St

Cal-Mor Circle

SW Morgan St

Beach Dr SW

48th Ave SW

47th Ave SW

Fauntleroy Way SW

SW Myrtle St

Samuel and Jessie Kenney Presbyterian Home

P U G E T   S O U N D

California Ave SW

35th Ave SW

SW Holden St

Bluff Trail

Fauntleroy Way SW

41st Ave SW

39th Ave SW

37th Ave SW

Colman Pool

LINCOLN PARK

SW Thistle St

South Beach Trail

Fauntleroy Ferry Terminal **finish**

ferry to Vashon Island

SW Barton St

0   200   400   600 yards
0   200   400   600 meters

35 LINCOLN Park TO FaUNTLeroy: THICK Trees aT THE EDGE OF THE SOUND

BOUNDARIES: **California Ave. SW, SW Graham St., Fauntleroy Way SW, and SW Henderson St.**
DISTANCE: **2½ miles**
DIFFICULTY: **Easy (almost all flat or downhill)**
PARKING: **Free street parking**
PUBLIC TRANSIT: **Metro routes #22, 54, and 128 stop at this route's start.**

A ferry ride to bucolic Vashon Island awaits at the end of a park stroll with grand Puget Sound views. Your walk starts with a residential stretch that's been upscaled several times in different decades, then continues past a sprawling Colonial-style retirement complex. Once in Lincoln Park you'll walk along the top of a bluff. You'll overlook both the Sound and a much quieter beach than Walk 33's Alki Beach. Then you'll descend to the beach and to an indoor saltwater pool, before your finale at the Fauntleroy ferry dock.

● Start on California Ave. SW, walking south from SW Graham St. To your right you first see a pair of delightfully rundown neighborhood businesses, Chuck & Sally's Tavern and the Short Stop convenience store. Halfway down this block, there's a tiny gem of a modern landscaped pocket park, Morgan Junction Park. Just beyond it are two neat little neighborhood eating and drinking spots, the upscale Beveridge Place Pub (named for the dead-end street just south of it) and the rock 'n' roll-themed Feed-back Lounge. The unusual round, eight-story apartment tower to your left is Cal-Mor Circle, operated as senior housing by the Seattle Housing Authority.

● Turn southwest on Fauntleroy Way SW. This street, which soon curves south, is a locale of solid single-family homes in a pleasing variety of sizes and styles. They include many '30s cottages and '50s ramblers, along with Craftsman bungalows (Seattle's standard housing stock, as you've seen from previous walks). This area, like much of West Seattle, didn't really take off as an upper-middle-class residential area until the post-World War II years. Many smaller homes were replaced at that time with larger successors. This trend was repeated during the 1990s–2000s boom.

- Turn west on SW Myrtle St. for one block, at the Samuel and Jessie Kenney Presbyterian Home, a massive retirement facility commonly called the Kenney. This sprawl of interconnected structures, built in a hodgepodge of styles between 1907 and 2003, somehow fits together architecturally.

- Turn south on 47th Ave. SW. To your left you can see the Kenney's original 1907 building. The elegant, cupola-topped brick structure is said to have been inspired by Philadelphia's Independence Hall. Two blocks later at 47th and SW Fontanelle St., the northeast corner of Lincoln Park is on your right.

- Enter Lincoln Park, walking southwest along a paved pathway. There are nearly five miles of trails within the 315-acre park; what follows is a simple way through. Follow the signs within the park onto the Bluff Trail, heading southwest toward (natch) a bluff overlooking the sound, the islands, and the Olympic Mountains. On parts of the trail you can look out toward the bluff. Some of these short clearings have benches for contemplation. On other parts of the trail, the view's hidden behind trees. On the whole trail, a fence separates you from the steepest descents. Want a more rigorous trek? Partake of the "exercise stations" installed along the trail.

- After the Bluff Trail curves southeast, follow a side path on your right to the South Beach Trail. It leads you downhill (sometimes steeply) toward (natch) the southern half of the park's beach. Once you reach the beach, take a right turn toward Colman Pool, at the point of this mini-peninsula. The outdoor, seasonally-open concrete pool uses filtered, heated saltwater. Even if you don't partake of the pool, you'll love the beach itself, with the waves, sand, and driftwood in front of you and the tree-covered bluff behind you.

- Backtrack the way you came on the paved South Beach Trail. Then continue farther on it, heading southeast along the shoreline. Take a paved path rising gently uphill from the beach, back into the park's interior, past a forest-themed jungle gym standing beneath tall madrona and Douglas-fir trees. Go east, out of the park and back to Fauntleroy.

- Resume walking south along Fauntleroy's east side. To your left, note some particularly snazzy brick Tudor-style houses.

Four blocks later you arrive at the Fauntleroy state ferry terminal. It's not a full-service passenger terminal like the downtown ferry depot (Walk 7), but rather a toll booth and a ramp toward the dock.

● From here you can take a ferry to Vashon Island or to Southworth on the Kitsap Peninsula. Vashon is a lovely countryside retreat bustling with farmers' markets and produce stands in the summertime. But be warned: The area immediately beyond the Vashon ferry dock is what bicyclists call a "chilly hilly," very steep for a long way. Metro routes #118 and 119 (Monday through Saturday only) can take you on a car-free scenic loop around the island.

● To return to this walk's start you can catch a #54 bus on the east side of Fauntleroy, across from the terminal.

CONNECTING THE WALKS

This walk ends three-quarters of a mile south of Walk 32's start.

POINTS OF INTEREST

Morgan Junction Park seattle.gov/parks, California Ave. SW and SW Beveridge Pl.

Beveridge Place Pub beveridgeplacepub.com, 6413 California Ave. SW

Feedback Lounge feedbacklounge.net, 6451 California Ave. SW, 206-453-3259

Cal-Mor Circle 6420 California Ave. SW

The Kenney thekenney.org, 7125 Fauntleroy Way SW, 206-937-2800

Lincoln Park seattle.gov/parks, 8011 Fauntleroy Way SW

Fauntleroy Ferry Terminal wsdot.wa.gov/ferries, 4829 SW Barton St.

route summary

1. Start on California Ave. SW, walking south from SW Graham St.
2. Turn southwest on Fauntleroy Way SW, which bends south.
3. Turn west on SW Myrtle St.
4. Turn south on 47th Ave. SW.
5. At 47th's end, enter Lincoln Park. Follow a main trail southwest to the beach at Colman Pool.
6. Turn southeast and inland, leaving the park.
7. Return to Fauntleroy, heading south to the Fauntleroy ferry terminal.

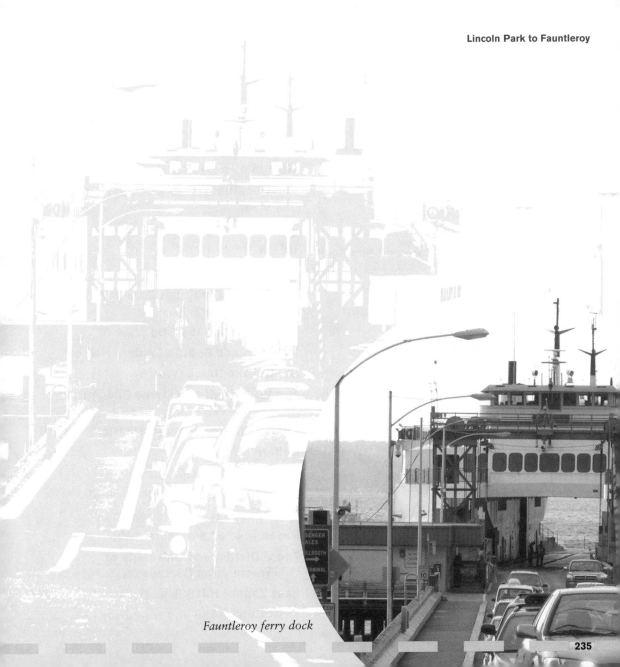

Fauntleroy ferry dock

Appendix 1: WALKS BY THEME

The walks below have at least one major component that fits the theme.

ARCHITECTURE

Pioneer Square (Walk 1)

Downtown: The Retail Core and Financial District (Walk 2)

Downtown: Off the Grid (Walk 3)

Pike Place Market and First Avenue (Walk 4)

Belltown and Seattle Center (Walk 5)

South Lake Union (Walk 6)

The Waterfront and Myrtle Edwards Park (Walk 7)

Discovery Park to Ballard Locks (Walk 10)

Chinatown-International District (Walk 11)

SoDo Industrial District (Walk 12)

Wallingford to Roosevelt (Walk 15)

The U District and University of Washington Campus (Walk 19)

Fairview and Eastlake (Walk 22)

East Capitol Hill (Walk 24)

West Capitol Hill and Broadway (Walk 25)

Pike-Pine (Walk 26)

First Hill (Walk 27)

Georgetown (Walk 31)

West Seattle: The Junction to Admiral (Walk 32)

THE ARTS

Pioneer Square (Walk 1)

Downtown: The Retail Core and Financial District (Walk 2)

Downtown: Off the Grid (Walk 3)

Belltown and Seattle Center (Walk 5)

South Lake Union (Walk 6)

The Waterfront and Myrtle Edwards Park (Walk 7)

Chinatown-International District (Walk 11)

Ballard (Walk 13)

Fremont (Walk 14)

Wallingford to Roosevelt (Walk 15)

Phinney Ridge and Greenwood (Walk 17)

Ravenna and Laurelhurst (Walk 18)

The U District and University of Washington Campus (Walk 19)

East Capitol Hill (Walk 24)

West Capitol Hill and Broadway (Walk 25)

Pike-Pine (Walk 26)

First Hill (Walk 27)

Central District (Walk 28)

Columbia City to Leschi (Walk 29)

Georgetown (Walk 31)

West Seattle: The Junction to Admiral (Walk 32)

Classic Seattle Neighborhoods

Pioneer Square (Walk 1)

Pike Place Market and First Avenue (Walk 4)

Belltown and Seattle Center (Walk 5)

South Lake Union (Walk 6)

Queen Anne Hill (Walk 8)

Magnolia (Walk 9)

Chinatown-International District (Walk 11)

Ballard (Walk 13)

Fremont (Walk 14)

Wallingford to Roosevelt (Walk 15)

Green Lake (Walk 16)

Phinney Ridge and Greenwood (Walk 17)

The U District and University of Washington Campus (Walk 19)

Madrona and Madison Park (Walk 21)

Fairview and Eastlake (Walk 22)

East Capitol Hill (Walk 24)

West Capitol Hill and Broadway (Walk 25)

Pike-Pine (Walk 26)

First Hill (Walk 27)

Central District (Walk 28)

Columbia City to Leschi (Walk 29)

Georgetown (Walk 31)

West Seattle: The Junction to Admiral (Walk 32)

Alki (Walk 33)

Dining and Entertainment

Pioneer Square (Walk 1)

Downtown: The Retail Core and Financial District (Walk 2)

Pike Place Market and First Avenue (Walk 4)

Belltown and Seattle Center (Walk 5)

South Lake Union (Walk 6)

The Waterfront and Myrtle Edwards Park (Walk 7)

Queen Anne Hill (Walk 8)

Magnolia (Walk 9)

Discovery Park to Ballard Locks (Walk 10)

Chinatown-International District (Walk 11)

SoDo Industrial District (Walk 12)

Ballard (Walk 13)

Fremont (Walk 14)

Wallingford to Roosevelt (Walk 15)

HISTOrY

INDUSTrY

Ballard (Walk 13)

Fremont (Walk 14)

Fairview and Eastlake (Walk 22)

Pike-Pine (Walk 26)

Georgetown (Walk 31)

West Marginal Way (Walk 34)

THe MUSIC SCeNe

Pioneer Square (Walk 1)

Belltown and Seattle Center (Walk 5)

South Lake Union (Walk 6)

Chinatown-International District (Walk 11)

SoDo Industrial District (Walk 12)

Ballard (Walk 13)

Fremont (Walk 14)

Wallingford to Roosevelt (Walk 15)

Ravenna and Laurelhurst (Walk 18)

The U District and University of
Washington Campus (Walk 19)

West Capitol Hill and Broadway (Walk 25)

Pike-Pine (Walk 26)

Georgetown (Walk 31)

West Seattle: The Junction to Admiral
(Walk 32)

ParKS

Pioneer Square (Walk 1)

Downtown: Off the Grid (Walk 3)

Belltown and Seattle Center (Walk 5)

South Lake Union (Walk 6)

The Waterfront and Myrtle Edwards Park
(Walk 7)

Queen Anne Hill (Walk 8)

Magnolia (Walk 9)

Discovery Park to Ballard Locks (Walk 10)

Fremont (Walk 14)

Wallingford to Roosevelt (Walk 15)

Green Lake (Walk 16)

Phinney Ridge and Greenwood (Walk 17)

Ravenna and Laurelhurst (Walk 18)

The U District and University of
Washington Campus (Walk 19)

Foster Island and the Arboretum (Walk
20)

Madrona and Madison Park (Walk 21)

Interlaken and Montlake (Walk 23)

East Capitol Hill (Walk 24)

Columbia City to Leschi (Walk 29)

Rainier Beach and Kubota Garden (Walk 30)

Georgetown (Walk 31)

West Marginal Way (Walk 34)

Lincoln Park to Fauntleroy (Walk 35)

Views

Pioneer Square (Walk 1)

Belltown and Seattle Center (Walk 5)

South Lake Union (Walk 6)

The Waterfront and Myrtle Edwards Park (Walk 7)

Queen Anne Hill (Walk 8)

Magnolia (Walk 9)

Discovery Park to Ballard Locks (Walk 10)

Fremont (Walk 14)

The U District and University of Washington Campus (Walk 19)

Foster Island and the Arboretum (Walk 20)

Madrona and Madison Park (Walk 21)

Fairview and Eastlake (Walk 22)

Interlaken and Montlake (Walk 23)

East Capitol Hill (Walk 24)

Pike-Pine (Walk 26)

Columbia City to Leschi (Walk 29)

Rainier Beach and Kubota Garden (Walk 30)

West Seattle: The Junction to Admiral (Walk 32)

Alki (Walk 33)

West Marginal Way (Walk 34)

Lincoln Park to Fauntleroy (Walk 35)

Water

Pioneer Square (Walk 1)

South Lake Union (Walk 6)

The Waterfront and Myrtle Edwards Park (Walk 7)

Queen Anne Hill (Walk 8)

Magnolia (Walk 9)

Discovery Park to Ballard Locks (Walk 10)

Ballard (Walk 13)

Fremont (Walk 14)

Green Lake (Walk 16)

The U District and University of Washington Campus (Walk 19)

Foster Island and the Arboretum (Walk 20)

Madrona and Madison Park (Walk 21)

Fairview and Eastlake (Walk 22)

Columbia City to Leschi (Walk 29)

Rainier Beach and Kubota Garden (Walk 30)

Alki (Walk 33)

West Marginal Way (Walk 34)

Lincoln Park to Fauntleroy (Walk 35)

Appendix 2 POINTS OF INTEREST

architectural and Historical Landmarks

Admiral Theater farawayentertainment.com/admiral.html, 2343 California Ave. SW, 206-938-0360 (Walk 32)

Alexander Pantages House 1117 36th Ave. E. (Walk 21)

Alki Homestead Restaurant 2717 61st Ave. SW (Walk 33)

Alki Point Lighthouse uscg.mil/history/weblighthouses/LHWA.asp, 3201 Alki Ave. SW, 206-841-3519 (Walk 33)

Anhalt Apartments 1005 E. Roy St. (Walk 25)

Ballard (Hiram M. Chittenden) Locks www.nws.usace.army.mil, 3015 NW 54th St., 206-783-7059 (Walk 10)

Bush School bush.edu, 405 36th Ave. E., 206-322-7978 (Walk 21)

Cal-Mor Circle 6420 California Ave. SW (Walk 35)

Calvary Catholic Cemetery acc-seattle.com/cemeteries/calvary.html, 5041 35th Ave. NE, 206-522-0996 (Walk 18)

College Inn collegeinnseattle.com, 4000 University Way NE, 206-634-2307 (Walk 19)

Colman Building 811 1st Ave. (Walk 3)

Columbia City Theater columbiacitytheater.com, 4918 Rainier Ave. S., 206-723-0088 (Walk 29)

Columbia Funeral Home columbiafuneralhome.com, 4567 Rainier Ave. S., 206-722-1100 (Walk 29)

Daniels Recital Hall recitalhall.fifthandcolumbia.com, 811 5th Ave., 425-922-6810 (Walk 2)

Discovery Park Visitor Center seattle.gov/parks, 3801 W. Government Way, 206-386-4236 (Walk 10)

Doubletree Arctic Club Hotel doubletree.hilton.com, 700 3rd Ave., 206-340-0340 (Walk 1)

Epiphany Parish of Seattle epiphanyseattle.org, 1805 38th Ave., 206-324-2573 (Walk 21)

Experience Music Project and Science Fiction Museum empsfm.org, 325 5th Ave. N., 877-EMP-SFM1 (Walk 5)

Fairmont Olympic Hotel fairmont.com/seattle, 411 University St., 206-621-1700 (Walk 2)

5th Avenue Theatre 5thavenue.org, 1326 5th Ave., 206-625-1900 (Walk 2)

Floating Homes Association seattlefloatinghomes.org, 2329 Fairview Ave. E., 206-325-1132 (Walk 22)

Fremont Bridge seattle.gov/transportation/bridges, Fremont Ave. N. south of N. Northlake Way (Walk 14)

Garfield High School ghs.seattleschools.org, 400 23rd Ave., 206-252-2270 (Walk 28)

Gas Works Park seattle.gov/parks, 2101 N. Northlake Way (Walk 14)

Georgetown PowerPlant Museum nps.gov/history/nr/travel/seattle/s35.htm, 6605 13th Ave. S., 206-763-2542 (Walk 31)

Good Shepherd Center historicseattle.org/projects/gsc.aspx, 4649 Sunnyside Ave. N. (Walk 15)

Harvard Exit Theater landmarktheatres.com, 807 E. Roy St., 206-781-5755 (Walk 25)

I-90 Overpass and Bike Tunnel traillink.com/trail/the-i-90-trail.aspx, Lake Washington Blvd. S. at S. Day St. (Walk 29)

Immaculate Conception Church immaculateconceptionseattle.org, 820 18th Ave., 206-322-5970 (Walk 28)

Inscape inscapearts.org, 815 Airport Way S., 206-257-3022 (Walk 11)

The Kenney thekenney.org, 7125 Fauntleroy Way SW, 206-937-2800 (Walk 35)

King Street Station seattle.gov/transportation/kingstreet.htm, 303 S. Jackson St., 206-382-4125 (Walk 1)

Klondike Gold Rush National Historical Park nps.gov/klse, 319 2nd Ave. S., 206-220-4240 (Walk 1)

Lake View Cemetery lakeviewcemeteryassociation.com, 1554 15th Ave. E., 206-322-1582 (Walk 24)

Langston Hughes Performing Arts Center seattle.gov/parks/centers/Langston.htm, 104 17th Ave. S., 206-684-4758 (Walk 28)

Log House Museum loghousemuseum.info, 3003 61st Ave. SW 206-938-5293 (Walk 33)

Seattle Tower 1218 3rd Ave. (Walk 3)

Seward School and Rogers Playground topsk8.org, 2500 Franklin Ave. E. (Walk 22)

Shafer Baillie Mansion sbmansion.com, 907 14th Ave. E., 206-322-4654 (Walk 24)

Smith Tower smithtower.com, 506 2nd Ave., 206-622-4004 (Walk 1)

Sorrento Hotel hotelsorrento.com, 900 Madison St., 206-343-6156 (Walk 27)

Space Needle spaceneedle.com, Broad St., 206-905-2100 (Walk 5)

St. James Cathedral stjames-cathedral.org, 804 9th Ave., 206-622-3559 (Walk 27)

St. Mark's Episcopal Cathedrai saintmarks.org, 1245 10th Ave. E., 206-323-0300 (Walk 25)

St. Spiridon Orthodox Cathedral saintspiridon.org, 400 Yale Ave. N. (Walk 6)

Sears at Starbucks Center sears.com, 76 S. Lander St., 206-344-4835 (Walk 12)

Stimson-Green Mansion stimsongreen.com, 1204 Minor Ave., 206-524-4918 (Walk 27)

Suzzallo Library lib.washington.edu/suzzallo, UW Central Plaza, 206-543-0242 (Walk 19)

Swedish Medical Center: Cherry Hill Campus swedish.org, 500 17th Ave., 206-320-2000 (Walk 28)

Town Hall Seattle townhallseattle.org, 1119 8th Ave., 206-652-4255 (Walk 27)

University of Washington Visitors Center washington.edu/discover/visit, 4060 George Washington Lane, 206-543-9198 (Walk 19)

Urban League of Metropolitan Seattle urbanleague.org, 105 14th Ave., 206-461-3792 (Walk 28)

Volunteer Park Conservatory volunteerparkconservatory.org, 1402 E. Galer St., 206-322-4112 (Walk 24)

Washington Hall washingtonhall.org, 153 14th Ave., 206-622-6952 (Walk 28)

Washington Pioneer Hall wapioneers.org, 1642 43rd Ave. (Walk 21)

Washington State Convention and Trade Center wsctc.com, 7th Ave. and Pike St. (Walk 2)

West Point Lighthouse foot of Utah Ave. in Discovery Park, 206-386-4236 (Walk 10)

West Seattle High School westseattlehs.seattleschools.org, 3000 California Ave. SW (Walk 32)

Westin Seattle starwoodhotels.com/westin/seattle, 1900 5th Ave., 206-728-1000 (Walk 5)

ZymoGenetics zymogenetics.com, 1201 Eastlake Ave. E. (Walk 22)

CHUrCHes

Admiral Congregational United Church of Christ admiralchurch.org, 4320 SW Hill St., 206-932-2928 (Walk 32)

All Pilgrims Christian Church allpilgrims.org, 500 Broadway E., 206-322-0487 (Walk 25)

Blessed Sacrament Church blessed-sacrament.org, 5041 9th Ave. NE, 206-546-3020 (Walk 15)

Duwamish Longhouse and Cultural Center duwamishtribe.org, 4705 West Marginal Way SW, 206-431-1582 (Walk 34)

Epiphany Parish of Seattle epiphanyseattle.org, 1805 38th Ave., 206-324-2573 (Walk 21)

Episcopal Church of the Ascension ascensionseattle.org, 2330 Viewmont Way W., 206-283-3967 (Walk 9)

First AME Church fameseattle.org, 1522 14th Ave., 206-324-3664 (Walk 26)

First Covenant Church firstcovenantseattle.org, 400 E. Pike St., 206-322-7411 (Walk 26)

Immaculate Conception Church immaculateconceptionseattle.org, 820 18th Ave., 206-322-5970 (Walk 28)

Immanuel Lutheran Church immanuelseattle.org, 1215 Thomas St. (Walk 6)

Magnolia Lutheran Church magnolialutheranchurch.com, 2414 31st Ave. W., 206-284-0155 (Walk 9)

Mars Hill Church marshillchurch.org, 1401 NW Leary Way (Walk 13)

Paradise of Praise Church paradiseofpraise.org, 1316 SW Holden St., 206-764-1053 (Walk 34)

Plymouth Church Seattle plymouthchurchseattle.org, 1217 6th Ave., 206-622-4865 (Walk 3)

Sakya Monastery sakya.org, 108 NW 83rd St., 206-789-2573 (Walk 17)

Seattle Church of Christ seattlechurchofchrist.org, 2555 8th Ave. W., 425-407-0582 (Walk 8)

Seattle First Baptist Church seattlefirstbaptist.org, 1111 Harvard Ave., 206-325-6051 (Walk 27)

Seattle University seattleu.edu, 901 12th Ave., 206-296-6000 (Walk 27)

St. Alphonsus Parish stalphonsus-sea.org, 5816 15th Ave. NW (Walk 13)

St. Demetrios Greek Orthodox Church saintdemetrios.com, 2100 Boyer Ave. E., 206-325-4347 (Walk 23)

St. James Cathedral stjames-cathedral.org, 804 9th Ave., 206-622-3559 (Walk 27)

St. John the Evangelist Catholic Church stjohnsea.org, 121 N. 80th St., 782-2810 (Walk 17)

St. Mark's Episcopal Cathedrai saintmarks.org, 1245 10th Ave. E., 206-323-0300 (Walk 25)

St. Nicholas Russian Orthodox Cathedral saintnicholascathedral.org, 1714 13th Ave. E., 206-322-9387 (Walk 24)

St. Paul's Episcopal Church stpaulseattle.org, 15 Roy St., 206-282-0786 (Walk 8)

St. Spiridon Orthodox Cathedral saintspiridon.org, 400 Yale Ave. N. (Walk 6)

Temple De Hirsch Sinai tdhs-nw.org, 1511 E. Pike St., 206-323-8486 (Walk 26)

Trinity Episcopal Church trinityseattle.com, 609 8th Ave., 206-624-5337 (Walk 27)

CULTUraL anD eDUCaTIONaL INSTITUTIONS

ACT Theatre acttheatre.org, 700 Union St., 206-292-7676 (Walk 3)

Alki Bathhouse and Art Studios seattle.gov/parks/arts/alkiart.htm, 2701 Alki Ave. SW, 206-684-7430 (Walk 33)

ArtsWest artswest.org, 4711 California Ave. SW, 206-938-0963 (Walk 32)

Ballard (Hiram M. Chittenden) Locks nws.usace.army.mil, 3015 NW 54th St., 206-783-7059 (Walk 10)

Burke Museum of Natural History and Culture washington.edu/burkemuseum, NE 45th St. and 17th Ave. NE, 206-543-5590 (Walk 19)

Bush School bush.edu, 405 36th Ave. E., 206-322-7978 (Walk 21)

Center for Wooden Boats cwb.org, 1010 Valley St., 206-382-2628 (Walk 6)

Cornish College of the Arts cornish.edu, 1000 Lenora St., 206-726-5151 (Walk 6)

Daybreak Star Indian Cultural Center unitedindians.org, northwest end of Discovery Park, 206-285-4425 (Walk 10)

Discovery Park Visitor Center seattle.gov/parks, 3801 W. Government Way, 206-386-4236 (Walk 10)

Duwamish Longhouse and Cultural Center duwamishtribe.org, 4705 West Marginal Way SW, 206-431-1582 (Walk 34)

826 Seattle 826seattle.org, 8414 Greenwood Ave. N., 206-725-2625 (Walk 17)

Experience Music Project and Science Fiction Museum empsfm.org, 325 5th Ave. N., 877-EMP-SFM1 (Walk 5)

Fremont Abbey Arts Center fremontabbey.org, 4272 Fremont Ave. N., 206-701-9270 (Walk 17)

Garfield High School ghs.seattleschools.org, 400 23rd Ave., 206-252-2270 (Walk 28)

Good Shepherd Center 4649 Sunnyside Ave. N. (Walk 15)

Henry Art Gallery henryart.org, 15th Ave. NE and NE 41st St, 206-543-2280 (Walk 19)

History House historyhouse.org, 709 N. 34th St., 206-675-8875 (Walk 14)

Inscape inscapearts.org, 815 Airport Way S., 206-257-3022 (Walk 11)

Klondike Gold Rush National Historical Park nps.gov/klse, 319 2nd Ave. S., 206-220-4240 (Walk 1)

Langston Hughes Performing Arts Center seattle.gov/parks/centers/Langston.htm, 104 17th Ave. S., 206-684-4758 (Walk 28)

Museum of History and Industry seattlehistory.org, 2700 24th Ave. E., 206-234-1126 (Walk 20)

Northwest Film Forum nwfilmforum.org, 1515 12th Ave., 206-329-2629 (Walk 26)

Olympic Sculpture Park seattleartmuseum.org, 2901 Western Ave., 206-654-3100 (Walk 7)

Pacific Science Center pacsci.org, 200 2nd Ave. N., 206-443-2001 (Walk 5)

Phinney Neighborhood Center phinneycenter.org, 6532 Phinney Ave. N., 206-783-2244 (Walk 17)

Photographic Center Northwest pcnw.org, 900 12th Ave., 206-720-7222 (Walk 27)

Pratt Fine Arts Center pratt.org, 1902 S. Main St., 206-328-2200 (Walk 28)

Rainier Beach High School 8815 Seward Park Ave. S. (Walk 30)

Rainier Valley Cultural Center seedseattle.org/seedarts, 3515 S. Alaska St., 206-725-7517 (Walk 29)

Raisbeck Performance Hall cornish.edu, 2015 Boren Ave., 206-726-5066 (Walk 6)

Richard Hugo House hugohouse.org, 1634 11th Ave., 206-322-7030 (Walk 26)

Seattle Aquarium seattleaquarium.org, 1483 Alaskan Way, 206-386-4320 (Walk 7)

Seattle Art Museum seattleartmuseum.org, 1300 1st Ave., 206-654-3100 (Walk 3)

Seattle Asian Art Museum seattleartmuseum.org, 1400 E. Prospect St., 206-654-3100 (Walk 24)

Seattle Center seattlecenter.com, 305 Harrison St., 206-684-7200 (Walk 5)

Seattle Central Community College seattlecentral.edu, 1701 Broadway, 206-587-3800 (Walk 26)

Seattle Central Library spl.org, 1000 4th Ave., 206-386-4636 (Walk 3)

Seattle Public Theater seattlepublictheater.org, 7312 West Green Lake Dr. N., 206-524-1300 (Walk 16)

Seattle University seattleu.edu, 901 12th Ave., 206-296-6000 (Walk 27)

Seward School and Rogers Playground topsk8.org, 2500 Franklin Ave. E. (Walk 22)

South Seattle Community College southseattle.edu, 6000 16th Ave. SW, 206-764-5300 (Walk 34)

Suzzallo Library lib.washington.edu/suzzallo, UW Central Plaza, 206-543-0242 (Walk 19)

University of Washington Visitors Center washington.edu/discover/visit, 4060 George Washington Lane, 206-543-9198 (Walk 19)

Volunteer Park Conservatory volunteerparkconservatory.org, 1402 E. Galer St., 206-322-4112 (Walk 24)

Washington Hall washingtonhall.org, 153 14th Ave., 206-622-6952 (Walk 28)

West Seattle High School westseattlehs.seattleschools.org, 3000 California Ave. SW (Walk 32)

Wing Luke Asian Museum wingluke.org, 707 S. King St., 206-623-5124 (Walk 11)

Woodland Park Zoo zoo.org, 5500 Phinney Ave. N., 206-548-2500 (Walk 17)

eaTING aND DrINKING

B&O Espresso b-oespresso.com, 204 Belmont Ave. E., 206-322-5028 (Walk 25)

Baranof 8549 Greenwood Ave. N., 206-782-9260 (Walk 17)

Beth's Cafe bethscafe.com, 7311 Aurora Ave. N., 206-782-5588 (Walk 16)

Beveridge Place Pub beveridgeplacepub.com, 6413 California Ave. SW (Walk 35)

Blue Moon Tavern bluemoonseattle.wordpress.com, 712 NE 45th St., 206-675-9116 (Walk 15)

Bush Garden bushgarden.net, 614 Maynard Ave. S., 206-682-6830 (Walk 11)

Cafe Racer caferacer.com, 5828 Roosevelt Way NE, 206-523-5282 (Walk 18)

Canterbury Ale & Eats 534 15th Ave. E., 206-322-3130 (Walk 24)

Chandler's Cove Marina 901 Fairview Ave. N. (Walk 6)

Charlestown Street Cafe charlestownchowder.com, 3800 California Ave. SW, 206-937-3800 (Walk 32)

Chelan Cafe 3527 Chelan Ave. SW, 206-932-7383 (Walk 12)

College Inn collegeinnseattle.com, 4000 University Way NE, 206-634-2307 (Walk 19)

Daniel's Restaurant Steakhouse and Bar schwartzbros.com/daniels.cfm, 200 Lake Washington Blvd., 206-329-4191 (Walk 29)

Dick's Drive-Ins dicksdrivein.com, 500 Queen Anne Ave. N. (Walk 8), 111 NE 45th St. (Walk 11), and 115 Broadway E. (Walk 25)

Eastlake Zoo Tavern eastlakezoo.com, 2301 Eastlake Ave. E., 206-329-3277 (Walk 22)

Easy Street Records and Cafe easystreetonline.com, 4559 California Ave. SW, 206-938-3279 (Walk 32)

Edgewater Hotel edgewaterhotel.com, 2411 Alaskan Way, Pier 67, 206-728-7000 (Walk 7)

Ezell's Famous Chicken ezellschicken.com, 501 23rd Ave., 206-324-4141 (Walk 28)

Feedback Lounge feedbacklounge.net, 6451 California Ave. SW, 206-453-3259 (Walk 35)

5 Point Cafe the5pointcafe.com, 415 Cedar St., 206-448-9993 (Walk 5)

14 Carrot Cafe 2305 Eastlake Ave. E., 206-324-1442 (Walk 22)

Fremont Coffee Company fremontcoffee.net, 459 N. 36th St., 206-632-3633 (Walk 14)

George & Dragon Pub georgeanddragonpub.com, 206 N. 36th St, 206-545-6864 (Walk 14)

Gim Wah 3418 W. McGraw St., 206-284-7000 (Walk 9)

Hale's Ales Pub halesbrewery.com, 4301 Leary Way NW, 206-706-1544 (Walk 14)

Heartland Cafe and Benbow Room heartlandcafeseattle.com, 4210 SW Admiral Way, 206-922-3313 (Walk 32)

Hi-Spot Cafe hispotcafe.com, 1410 34th Ave., 206-325-7905 (Walk 21)

Husky Deli huskydeli.com, 4721 California Ave. SW, 206-937-2810 (Walk 32)

Ivar's Acres of Clams ivars.com, Alaskan Way, Pier 54, 206-624-6852 (Walk 7)

Ivar's Salmon House ivars.com, 401 NE Northlake Way, 206-632-0767 (Walk 19)

Little Red Hen littleredhen.com, 7115 Woodlawn Ave. NE, 206-522-1168 (Walk 16)

Lockspot Cafe 3005 NW 54th St., 206-789-4865 (Walk 10)

Magnolia Village Pub magnolia-villagepub.com, 3221 W. McGraw St., 206-285-9756 (Walk 9)

Mike's Chili Parlor Tavern mikeschiliparlor.com, 1447 NW Ballard Way, 206-782-4641 (Walk 13)

Ozzie's Diner ozziesseattle.com, 105 W. Mercer St., 206-284-4618 (Walk 8)

Pacific Place pacificplaceseattle.com, 600 Pine St. (Walk 2)

Panama Hotel Tea & Coffee House panamahotel.net, 607 S. Main St., 206-515-4000 (Walk 11)

Pecos Pit BBQ 2260 1st Ave. S., 206-623-0629 (Walk 12)

Pepperdock Restaurant 2618 Alki Ave. SW, 206-935-1000 (Walk 33)

Peso's pesoskitchen.com, 605 Queen Anne Ave. N., 206-283-9353 (Walk 8)

Pike Place Market pikeplacemarket.org, 1st Ave. and Pike St., 206-682-7453 (Walk 4)

Portside Coffee 6720 West Marginal Way SW (Walk 34)

Red Mill Burgers at the Totem House redmillburgers.com, 3058 NW 54th St. (Walk 10)

Red Onion Tavern 4210 E. Madison St., 206-323-1611 (Walk 21)

Romio's Pizza romios-pizza.com, 3242 Eastlake Ave. E., 206-322-4453 (Walk 23)

Slim's Last Chance Chili Shack slimslastchance.com, 5506 1st Ave. S., 206-762-7900 (Walk 31)

Space Needle spaceneedle.com, 400 Broad St., 905-2100 (Walk 5)

Spud Fish & Chips spudfishandchips.com, 6860 East Green Lake Dr. N. (Walk 16) and 2666 Alki Ave. SW (Walk 33)

Tai Tung 659 S. King St., 206-622-7372 (Walk 11)

Targy's 600 W. Crockett St., 206-352-8882 (Walk 8)

13 Coins 13coins.com, 125 Boren Ave. N., 206-682-2513 (Walk 6)

Top Pot Doughnuts toppotdoughnuts.com, 2100 5th Ave. (Walk 5); 609 Summit Ave. E. (Walk 25)

Tractor Tavern tractortavern.com, 5213 Ballard Ave. NW, 206-789-3599 (Walk 13)

Upper Crust Bakery uppercrustseattle.com, 3204 W. McGraw St., 206-283-1003 (Walk 9)

Uwajimaya uwajimaya.com, 600 5th Ave. S., 206-624-6248 (Walk 11)

Vegetable Bin Polynesian Deli 8816 Martin Luther King Jr. Way S., 206-725-0543 (Walk 30)

Victrola Coffee and Art victrolacoffee.com, 411 15th Ave. E., 206-325-6520 (Walk 24)

Virginia Inn virginiainnseattle.com, 1937 1st Ave., 206-728-1937 (Walk 4)

Westlake Center westlakecenter.com, 400 Pine St. (Walk 2)

Zesto's Burger and Fish House zestosseattle.com, 6416 15th Ave. NW, 206-783-3350 (Walk 13)

ENTERTAINMENT AND NIGHTLIFE

ACT Theatre acttheatre.org, 700 Union St., 206-292-7676 (Walk 3)

Admiral Theater farawayentertainment.com/admiral.html, 2343 California Ave. SW, 206-938-0360 (Walk 32)

Broadway Performance Hall broadwayperfhall.com, 1625 Broadway, 206-325-3113 (Walk 26)

Central Cinema central-cinema.com, 1411 21st Ave., 206-686-6864 (Walk 28)

Can Can thecancan.com, 94 Pike St., 206-652-0832 (Walk 4)

Columbia City Theater columbiacitytheater.com, 4918 Rainier Ave. S., 206-723-0088 (Walk 29)

Daniels Recital Hall recitalhall.fifthandcolumbia.com, 811 5th Ave., 425-922-6810 (Walk 2)

Egyptian Theatre landmarktheatres.com, 805 E. Pine St., 206-720-4560 (Walk 26)

El Corazón elcorazonseattle.com, 109 Eastlake Ave E., 206-381-3094 (Walk 6)

5th Avenue Theatre 5thavenue.org, 1326 5th Ave., 206-625-1900 (Walk 2)

Hale's Ales Pub halesbrewery.com, 4301 Leary Way NW, 206-706-1544 (Walk 14)

Harvard Exit Theater landmarktheatres.com, 807 E. Roy St., 206-781-5755 (Walk 25)

Hec Edmundson Pavilion gohuskies.com, 3870 Montlake Blvd. NE, 206-543-2200 (Walk 19)

High Dive highdiveseattle.com, 513 N. 36th St., 206-632-9212 (Walk 14)

Langston Hughes Performing Arts Center seattle.gov/parks/centers/Langston.htm, 104 17th Ave. S., 206-684-4758 (Walk 28)

Moore Theatre stgpresents.org, 1932 2nd Ave., 206-443-1744 (Walk 5)

Nectar nectarlounge.com, 412 N. 36th St., 206-632-2020 (Walk 14)

Northwest Film Forum nwfilmforum.org, 1515 12th Ave., 206-329-2629 (Walk 26)

On the Boards ontheboards.org, 100 W. Roy St., 206-217-9886 (Walk 8)

Paramount Theater stgpresents.org, 911 Pine St., 206-467-5510 (Walk 2)

Qwest Field qwestfield.com, 800 Occidental Ave. S., 206-682-2900 (Walk 1)

Re-bar rebarseattle.com, 1114 Howell St., 206-223-9873 (Walk 6)

Safeco Field mariners.mlb.com, 1250 1st Ave. S., 206-346-4001 (Walk 12)

Seattle Public Theater seattlepublictheater.org, 7312 West Green Lake Dr. N., 206-524-1300 (Walk 16)

Showbox at the Market showboxonline.com, 1426 1st Ave., 206-628-3151 (Walk 4)

Slim's Last Chance Chili Shack slimslastchance.com, 5506 1st Ave. S., 206-762-7900 (Walk 31)

Sunset Tavern sunsettavern.com, 5433 Ballard Ave. NW, 206-784-4880 (Walk 13)

Teatro ZinZanni zinzanni.org, 222 Mercer St., 206-802-0015 (Walk 5)

The Crocodile thecrocodile.com, 2200 2nd Ave., 206-441-7416 (Walk 5)

Theatre Off Jackson theatreoffjackson.org, 409 7th Ave. S., 206-340-1049 (Walk 11)

Tractor Tavern tractortavern.com, 5213 Ballard Ave. NW, 206-789-3599 (Walk 13)

Washington Hall washingtonhall.org, 153 14th Ave., 206-622-6952 (Walk 28)

Galleries and Museums

ArtsWest artswest.org, 4711 California Ave. SW, 206-938-0963 (Walk 32)

Burke Museum of Natural History and Culture washington.edu/burkemuseum, NE 45th St. and 17th Ave. NE, 206-543-5590 (Walk 19)

Experience Music Project and Science Fiction Museum empsfm.org, 325 5th Ave. N., 877-EMP-SFM1 (Walk 5)

Frye Art Museum fryemuseum.org, 704 Terry Ave., 206-622-9250 (Walk 27)

Georgetown PowerPlant Museum nps.gov/history/nr/travel/seattle/s35.htm, 6605 13th Ave. S., 206-763-2542 (Walk 31)

Henry Art Gallery henryart.org, 15th Ave. NE and NE 41st St, 206-543-2280 (Walk 19)

Klondike Gold Rush National Historical Park nps.gov/klse, 319 2nd Ave. S., 206-220-4240 (Walk 1)

Log House Museum loghousemuseum.info, 3003 61st Ave. SW, 206-938-5293 (Walk 33)

Museum of Communications museumofcommunications.org, 7000 East Marginal Way S., 206-767-3012 (Walk 31)

Museum of Flight museumofflight.org, 9409 E. Marginal Way, 206-764-5700 (Walk 31)

Museum of History and Industry seattlehistory.org, 2700 24th Ave. E., 206-234-1126 (Walk 20)

Olympic Sculpture Park seattleartmuseum.org, 2901 Western Ave., 206-654-3100 (Walk 7)

Pacific Science Center pacsci.org, 200 2nd Ave. N., 206-443-2001 (Walk 5)

Photographic Center Northwest pcnw.org, 900 12th Ave., 206-720-7222 (Walk 27)

Seattle Art Museum seattleartmuseum.org, 1300 1st Ave., 206-654-3100 (Walk 3)

Seattle Asian Art Museum seattleartmuseum.org, 1400 E. Prospect St., 206-654-3100 (Walk 24)

Seattle Glassblowing Studio seattleglassblowing.com, 2227 5th Ave., 206-448-2181 (Walk 5)

Seattle Metropolitan Police Museum seametropolicemuseum.org, 317 3rd Ave. S., 206-748-9991 (Walk 1)

Wing Luke Asian Museum wingluke.org, 707 S. King St., 206-623-5124 (Walk 11)

HOTELS

College Inn collegeinnseattle.com, 4000 University Way NE, 206-634-2307 (Walk 19)

Doubletree Arctic Club Hotel doubletree.hilton.com, 700 3rd Ave., 206-340-0340 (Walk 1)

Edgewater Hotel edgewaterhotel.com, 2411 Alaskan Way, Pier 67, 206-728-7000 (Walk 7)

Fairmont Olympic Hotel fairmont.com/seattle, 411 University St., 206-621-1700 (Walk 2)

Four Seasons Hotel and Condos fourseasons.com/seattle, 99 Union St., 206-749-7000 (Walk 4)

Sorrento Hotel hotelsorrento.com, 900 Madison St., 206-343-6156 (Walk 27)

Westin Seattle starwoodhotels.com/westin/seattle, 1900 5th Ave., 206-728-1000 (Walk 5)

Parks

Alki Beach Park seattle.gov/parks, 1702 Alki Ave. SW (Walk 33)

Atlantic City Boat Ramp seattle.gov/parks/Boats/motorized.htm, 8702 Seward Park Ave. S., 206-684-7249 (Walk 30)

Ballard (Hiram M. Chittenden) Locks nws.usace.army.mil, 3015 NW 54th St., 206-783-7059 (Walk 10)

Beer Sheva Park seattle.gov/parks, 8650 55th Ave. S. (Walk 30)

Colman Park seattle.gov/parks, 1800 Lake Washington Blvd. S. (Walk 29)

Denny-Blaine Park seattle.gov/parks, 200 Lake Washington Blvd. E. (Walk 21)

Discovery Park Visitor Center seattle.gov/parks, 3801 W. Government Way, 206-386-4236 (Walk 10)

Ella Bailey Park seattle.gov/parks, 27th Ave. W. and W. Smith St. (Walk 9)

Freeway Park seattle.gov/parks, 700 Seneca St. (Walk 3)

Frink and Leschi Parks seattle.gov/parks, 398 Lake Washington Blvd. S. (Walk 29)

Gas Works Park seattle.gov/parks, 2101 N. Northlake Way (Walk 14)

Good Shepherd Center historicseattle.org/projects/gsc.aspx, 4649 Sunnyside Ave. N. (Walk 15)

Green Lake Park seattle.gov/parks, 7201 East Green Lake Dr. N. (Walk 16)

I-90 Overpass and Bike Tunnel traillink.com/trail/the-i-90-trail.aspx, Lake Washington Blvd. S. at S. Day St. (Walk 29)

Interlaken Park seattle.gov/parks, 2451 Delmar Ave. E. (Walk 23)

Kerry Park seattle.gov/parks, 211 W. Highland Dr. (Walk 8)

Klondike Gold Rush National Historical Park nps.gov/klse, 319 2nd Ave. S., 206-220-4240 (Walk 1)

Kobe Terrace seattle.gov/parks, 221 6th Ave. S. (Walk 11)

Kubota Garden kubota.org, 9817 55th Ave. S., 206-684-4584 (Walk 30)

Lincoln Park seattle.gov/parks, 8011 Fauntleroy Way SW (Walk 35)

Lynn Street Park seattle.gov/parks, Fairview Ave. E. and E. Lynn St. (Walk 22)

Madison Park seattle.gov/parks, E. Madison St. and E. Howe St. (Walk 21)

Magnolia Park seattle.gov/parks, 1461 Magnolia Blvd. W. (Walk 9)

Mini Mart City Park minimartcitypark.com, 6525 Ellis Ave. S., 206-722-2116 (Walk 31)

Montlake Playground and Community Center seattle.gov/parks, 1618 E. Calhoun St., 206-684-4736 (Walk 23)

Morgan Junction Park seattle.gov/parks, California Ave. SW and SW Beveridge Pl. (Walk 35)

Mt. Baker Rowing and Sailing Center mbrsc.org, 3800 Lake Washington Blvd. S., 206-386-1913 (Walk 29)

Myrtle Edwards Park seattle.gov/parks, 3130 Alaskan Way W., 206-684-4075 (Walk 7)

Occidental Park seattle.gov/parks, Occidental Ave. S. and S. Washington St. (Walk 1)

Olympic Sculpture Park seattleartmuseum.org, 2901 Western Ave., 206-654-3100 (Walk 7)

Oxbow Park seattle.gov/parks, 6425 Carleton Ave. S. (Walk 31)

Peace Park seattle.gov/parks, NE 40th St. and 9th Ave. NE (Walk 19)

Pioneer Square seattle.gov/parks, 1st Ave. and Yesler Way (Walk 1)

Plymouth Pillars Park seattle.gov/parks, Boren Ave. and Pike St. (Walk 26)

Rainier Beach Community Center and Playfield seattle.gov/parks/centers/rainierbeach.htm, 8825 Rainier Ave. S., 206-386-1925 (Walk 30)

Ravenna and Cowen Park seattle.gov/parks, 5849 15th Ave. NE, 206-548-2500 (Walk 18)

Roanoke Park seattle.gov/parks, 2409 10th Ave. E. (Walk 23)

Schmitz Preserve Park seattle.gov/parks, 5551 SW Admiral Way (Walk 32)

Seacrest Park seattle.gov/parks, 1660 Harbor Ave. SW (Walk 33)

Seattle Center seattlecenter.com, 305 Harrison St., 206-684-7200 (Walk 5)

Seattle Japanese Garden seattle.gov/parks, 1075 Lake Washington Blvd. E., 206-684-4725 (Walk 20)

Seward School and Rogers Playground topsk8.org, 2500 Franklin Ave. E. (Walk 22)

Terminal 105 Park portseattle.org, 4260 West Marginal Way SW (Walk 34)

Terminal 107 Park portseattle.org, 4700 West Marginal Way SW (Walk 34)

University of Washington Visitors Center washington.edu/discover/visit, 4060 George Washington Lane, 206-543-9198 (Walk 19)

UW Waterfront Activities Center depts.washington.edu/ima/IMA_wac.php, 3900 Montlake Blvd. NE, 206-534-9433 (Walk 20)

Viretta Park seattle.gov/parks, 39th Ave. E. and E. John St. (Walk 21)

Volunteer Park Conservatory volunteerparkconservatory.org, 1402 E. Galer St., 206-322-4112 (Walk 24)

Washington Park Arboretum depts.washington.edu/uwbg/gardens/wpa.shtml, 2300 Arboretum Dr. E., 206-543-8800 (Walk 20)

Waterfall Garden Park 219 2nd Ave. S. (Walk 1)

West Duwamish Greenbelt and Puget Park seattle.gov/parks, Highland Park Way SW and West Marginal Way SW (Walk 34)

Woodland Park Zoo zoo.org, 5500 Phinney Ave. N., 206-548-2500 (Walk 17)

SHOPPING

Archie McPhee archiemcpheeseattle.com, 1300 N. 45th St., 206-297-0240 (Walk 15)

Arundel Books arundelbookstores.com, 1001 1st Ave., 206-624-4442 (Walk 4)

Atomic Boys atomicboysseattle.com, 4311 SW Admiral Way, 206-938-3255 (Walk 32)

Big John's PFI bigjohnspfi.com, 1001 6th Ave. S., 206-682-2022 (Walk 11)

Burnt Sugar and Frankie Boutiques store.burntsugarfrankie.com, 601 N. 35th St., 206-545-0699 (Walk 14)

Chandler's Cove Marina 901 Fairview Ave. N. (Walk 6)

Cinema Books cinemabooks.net, 4753 Roosevelt Way NE, 206-547-7667 (Walk 15)

City Market 1722 Bellevue Ave., 206-323-1715 (Walk 25)

Costco costco.com, 4401 4th Ave. S., 206-674-1220 (Walk 12)

Easy Street Records and Cafe easystreetonline.com, 4559 California Ave. SW, 206-938-3279 (Walk 32)

Elliott Bay Book Co. elliottbaybook.com, 1521 10th Ave., 206-624-6600 (Walk 26)

European Vine Selections evswines.com, 522 15th Ave E., 206-323-3557 (Walk 24)

Fantagraphics Books fantagraphics.com, 1201 S. Vale St., 206-658-0110 (Walk 31)

Galway Traders galwaytraders.com, 7518 15th Ave. NW, 206-784-9343 (Walk 13)

Gasoline Alley Antiques gasolinealleyantiques.com, 6501 20th Ave. NE, 206-524-1606 (Walk 18)

Georgetown Records georgetownrecords.net, 1201 S. Vale St., 206-762-5638 (Walk 31)

Georgetown Trailer Park Mall georgetowntrailerpark.com, 947 Doris St. (Walk 31)

Gregg's Greenlake Cycle greggscycles.com, 7007 Woodlawn Ave. NE, 206-523-1822 (Walk 16)

Island Life island-life.com, 2909 1st Ave. S., 206-340-1212 (Walk 12)

Kobo at Higo koboseattle.com, 604 S. Jackson St., 206-381-3000 (Walk 11)

Magnolia's Bookstore 3206 W. McGraw St., 206-283-1062 (Walk 9)

Metsker Maps metskers.com, 1511 1st Ave., 206-623-8747 (Walk 4)

Not A Number Cards and Gifts notanumbergifts.com, 1905 N. 45th St., 206-784-0965 (Walk 15)

Pacific Galleries pacgal.com, 241 S. Lander St., 206-292-3999 (Walk 12)

Pacific Place pacificplaceseattle.com, 600 Pine St. (Walk 2)

Patrick's Fly Shop patricksflyshop.com, 2237 Eastlake Ave. E., 206-325-8988 (Walk 22)

Pete's Wines peteswineshop.com, 58 E. Lynn St., 206-322-2660 (Walk 22)

Pike Place Market pikeplacemarket.org, 1st Ave. and Pike St., 206-682-7453 (Walk 4)

Pretty Parlor prettyparlor.com, 110 Summit Ave. E., 206-405-2883 (Walk 25)

REI rei.com/stores, 222 Yale Ave. N., 206-223-1944 (Walk 6)

The RE Store re-store.org, 1440 NW 52nd St., 206-297-9119 (Walk 13)

Scandinavian Specialties scanspecialties.com, 6719 15th Ave. NW, 206-784-7020 (Walk 13)

Scarecrow Video scarecrow.com, 5030 Roosevelt Way NE, 206-524-8554 (Walk 15)

Sears at Starbucks Center sears.com, 76 S. Lander St., 206-344-4835 (Walk 12)

Third Place Books ravenna.thirdplacebooks.com, 6504 20th Ave. NE, 206-736-5009 (Walk 18)

Trading Musician tradingmusician.com, 5908 Roosevelt Way NE, 206-522-6707 (Walk 18)

University Book Store bookstore.washington.edu, 4326 University Way NE, 206-548-2500 (Walk 19)

University Village uvillage.com, 2673 NE University Village Way, 206-523-0622 (Walk 18)

Uwajimaya uwajimaya.com, 600 5th Ave. S., 206-624-6248 (Walk 11)

Vegetable Bin Polynesian Deli 8816 Martin Luther King Jr. Way S., 206-725-0543 (Walk 30)

Westlake Center westlakecenter.com, 400 Pine St. (Walk 2)

FurTHer reaDING

BOOKS

A Guide to Architecture in Washington State by Sally B. Woodbridge and Roger Montgomery. Seattle: University of Washington Press, 1980. The many strains of late-19th- and 20th-century design, as applied to the built environment.

The Fountain and the Mountain: The University of Washington Campus in Seattle by Norman J. Johnson. Seattle: Documentary Media, 1995–2006. Gorgeous coffee-table tribute to the UW and its fabulous grounds.

Meet Me at the Center: The Story of Seattle Center by Don Duncan. Seattle: Seattle Center Foundation, 1992. The center, the World's Fair that spawned it, and how the city has celebrated itself.

The Pike Place Market: People, Politics, and Produce by Alice Shorett and Murray Morgan. Seattle: Pacific Search Press, 1982. The politics, economics, and design behind the market and its 1970s revamp.

Seattle & King County Timeline by Walt Crowley and the HistoryLink Staff. Seattle: University of Washington Press, 2001. A slim volume jam-packed with pictures of and fun facts about the Jet City.

Seattle and the Demons of Ambition by Fred Moody. New York: St. Martin's Press, 2003. A look back at Seattle's cravings to become "world class," from its pioneer days to the dot-com era.

Seattle Architecture by Maureen R. Elenga. Seattle: University of Washington Press, 2008. From Pioneer Square to Seattle Center, downtown Seattle's major structures and how they got designed and built.

Shaping Seattle Architecture: A Historical Guide to the Architects edited by Jeffrey Karl Ochsner. Seattle: University of Washington Press, 2003. The people behind Seattle's greatest structures.

Wet and Wired by Randy Hodgkins and Steve McLellan. Dallas: Taylor Trade Publishing, 2000. A breezy introductory course in Northwest pop culture.

WEBSITES

Arcade, www.arcadejournal.com. A sounding board for the Northwest design community.

HistoryLink, www.historylink.org. An ever-growing online encyclopedia of Seattle and Northwest history.

Publicola, www.publicola.net. An inside-the-sausage-factory look at how Seattle politics and civic planning really work.

Seattle Architecture Foundation, www.seattlearchitecture.org. Tours and educational programs about the city's past and its future.

Seattle Dream Homes, www.seattledreamhomes.com. Much more than a real-estate sales site, with sections on artistic, historic, and "roadside" Seattle.

A Year of Seattle Parks, www.yearofseattleparks.blogspot.com. Linnea Westerlind visited all 406 Seattle parks in one year. This is her story.

INDEX

(*Italicized* page numbers indicate photos.)

aBOUT THe auTHor

Clark Humphrey has done a lot of things in a lot of years, almost all of them within the Jet City. He's walked his way through every Seattle neighborhood except the gated Broadmoor. Clark's a former staff writer with *The Stranger* and *The Comics Journal,* and a former book reviewer for *The Seattle Times*. His previous books include *Loser: The Real Seattle Music Story* (Feral House), and *Vanishing Seattle* and *Seattle's Belltown* (both Arcadia Publishing). His ongoing thoughts about the city and its growth can be found at miscmedia.com.

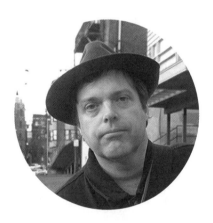